Beyond Precision

Beyond Precision

How AI Personalizes Your Care—Without Understanding Who You Are

Elias Wren

Mindful Pages

Published in 2025

ISBN: 9789371770439 (PB)
ISBN: 9789371774932 (eBook)

Published by

Mindful Pages
Imprint of Alpha Editions LLC
312 W. 2nd St #1834
Casper, WY 82601, USA

This book was developed using advanced writing tools to support the drafting and ideation process. All content has been thoughtfully curated, refined, and reviewed to ensure quality and relevance.

Content

Introduction
Illusion of Understanding

The allure is undeniable: a future where healthcare sheds its one-size-fits-all cloak and becomes exquisitely personal. Imagine medicine that knows you—your genes, your rhythms, your vulnerabilities—so well it can foresee illness before a symptom dares to surface. A world where treatment isn't assigned by protocol but chosen, almost intuitively, to fit the intricate contours of your biology. Artificial intelligence, the prophets say, will deliver us from the frailties of human judgement and the strain of overloaded systems. It will diagnose with clarity, prescribe with precision, and—most beguiling of all—anticipate our needs before we know them ourselves.

Yet beneath this polished vision lies something deeply unsettling. The machines that promise to revolutionise care do not, in any meaningful sense, understand us. They cannot fathom fear, or hope, or the quiet ache of uncertainty that accompanies a diagnosis. They do not notice hesitation in a trembling voice, nor the pain disguised in a patient's polite nod. To AI, a human being is structure and signal—never story. It perceives probabilities, not persons. It parses patterns but is blind to meaning. And still, this mechanical form of "understanding" is rapidly becoming the new benchmark of intelligence in medicine.

This, then, is the contradiction at the heart of *Beyond Precision*.

The book is no technophobic manifesto. Nor is it a sentimental ode to intuition. Rather, it is a sober inquiry into the widening gap between what algorithms predict and what people actually live through. It challenges the seductive idea that more data naturally means better care—a notion that, while persuasive, is philosophically fragile and practically treacherous. For all its sophistication, AI in healthcare remains strikingly blind to the messy, irreducible complexity of being human. If that blindness goes unexamined, we risk swapping yesterday's exclusions for tomorrow's—more hidden, perhaps, but no less harmful.

To see how this matters, we must recognise the nature of the transformation underway. Medicine is not merely acquiring new tools; it is adopting a new logic. Care, once grounded in interpretation, dialogue, and moral discernment, is being recast as a matter of optimisation. The patient ceases to be a subject of concern and becomes a site of calculation. Their story dissolves into data; their symptoms become signals; their preferences, probabilities.

Here is where illusion begins to harden into belief: that a system may be deeply personalised without being remotely personalist. That bespoke treatment can exist without genuine understanding. That a statistical model might rival, or even replace, the steady gaze of a clinician who has not only read a patient's chart but listened to their fears.

To be fair, this is not an attack on AI's competence. Its diagnostic precision is often astonishing—identifying tumours, predicting sepsis, managing triage with a speed and accuracy beyond human capacity. The point, however, is subtler: accuracy is not understanding. Prediction is not care. To conflate them is to usher in a cultural and ethical shift of profound consequence.

Too often, discourse around AI in medicine lurches between utopian optimism and dystopian dread. *Beyond Precision* seeks another path—anchored in reality, guided by lived experience, and enriched by the multiple disciplines that converge in the act of caring. It draws insight from medicine and data science, yes, but also from philosophy, design, anthropology, and ethics. The question is not simply what these technologies *can* do, but what they *should* do—and for whom.

There is, undeniably, promise here. AI's power to tailor interventions, uncover hidden correlations, and expand access to care is real. Yet this progress comes at a conceptual cost: the gradual erasure of the patient as a speaking subject. In its place emerges a quieter paradigm—one that acts *for* people, not *with* them. The danger is not that AI will replace doctors, but that it will redefine what it means to be a patient, and, more gravely, what it means to be cared for.

We can already see this shift in motion. Think of wearable trackers that whisper advice while subtly recalibrating our sense of normal. Or diagnostic systems that perform brilliantly on curated datasets but falter when faced with an actual human body—messy, noncompliant, inconveniently unique. Or triage algorithms that prioritise efficiency over empathy, calculating benefit while quietly encoding social bias. These are not future hypotheticals. They are happening now—in hospitals, clinics, even living rooms.

What unites these examples is not malice, but mismatch. The logic of machines and the lifeworld of humans simply do not align. The harm appears not in dramatic failures but in quiet misrecognitions: the patient whose pain goes unrecorded because it lies outside the data model; the doctor who second-guesses her own instincts in deference to a screen; the health system that relies on predictive tools without questioning whose futures they truly serve.

Hence, *Beyond Precision* poses a set of uncomfortable but necessary questions. What do we lose when we privilege pattern over presence? Can ethical care survive in systems designed for prediction rather than understanding? How do we ensure that technology amplifies rather than erodes the human core of medicine? And most crucially: what kind of healthcare system are we building—not just in outcomes, but in values?

These questions are not academic niceties. They press on every aspect of healthcare, from policy and software design to bedside interaction and professional training. They compel us to act not merely as consumers of innovation but as custodians of care. For AI, far from lessening our responsibility, intensifies it.

That responsibility begins with better questions—not merely about what works efficiently, but what matters deeply. About dignity as much as data. About personhood, not just personalisation.

In the pages ahead, we will examine where AI-driven precision succeeds and where it falters. We will probe the seductive logic of optimisation and the hidden costs it conceals. We will hear from doctors negotiating the uneasy border between intuition and automation, from patients navigating the ambiguities of algorithmic medicine, and from researchers wrestling with the limits of their own models.

We will trace the long drift from interpretation to computation, from human judgement to quantified certainty. We will confront the biases that stain our datasets, the quiet violence of systems that confuse silence with consent. We will explore how design might protect complexity rather than crush it, how institutions might defend humaneness rather than sacrifice it to scale, and how citizens—patients, practitioners, policymakers alike—can reclaim a say in the architecture of care.

This is not a book against technology. It is a book against reduction.

Because precision, as we shall see, is not synonymous with care. And if care is to survive, we must learn to look past precision—toward the fragile, astonishing, unquantifiable human being at its centre.

Chapter 1
The Personalized Mirage

Step into any contemporary healthcare conference, leaf through a cutting-edge medical technology journal, or scroll through the sleek marketing copy of a biotech start-up, and you'll hear the same confident chorus: the future is personalised. No longer will illness be treated by type, but by code—each of us mapped through our genomes, monitored through wearables, interpreted by algorithms, and prescribed with near-mathematical precision. Personalisation, they insist, isn't merely an improvement to medicine; it's a full-blown transformation. The era of generic treatments and uniform protocols is drawing to a close. In its place stands a new order, one powered by artificial intelligence and dedicated to tailoring healthcare to the finest molecular and behavioural detail.

It's an easy dream to buy into. Who wouldn't prefer medicine that recognises them as an individual rather than a data point? The notion that care might be designed to fit *you*—your chemistry, your habits, your particular vulnerabilities—is irresistible. And the vocabulary surrounding it is deliberately seductive: precision, optimisation, customisation. Words borrowed from luxury markets, now repurposed for the clinic. They speak to more than medical progress; they evoke a cultural promise—that individuality itself can be technologically perfected.

Yet beneath this confident rhetoric lies a quieter, more searching question: what does it mean for medicine to "know" us? When does prediction cross the threshold into understanding? And can a system that perceives only data ever be said to perceive a person?

That is where this chapter begins.

We begin by confronting the central myth that underpins AI-driven personalisation—the idea that an abundance of data, combined with sufficient computational power, will naturally yield superior care. It's a belief built on real triumphs: genomics can now identify genetic risks with astonishing precision; wearable devices produce unbroken streams of physiological data; algorithms can detect early signs of disease in scans faster than human experts. The achievements are undeniable. Yet the leap from technical capability to the claim of true personalisation is not an inevitable one—it's a narrative choice, shaped by human longing as much as by machine capacity.

To appreciate what AI-based personalisation actually does, we must first grasp its operational logic. Predictive systems in healthcare do not *understand* patients as such; they identify statistical regularities across massive datasets—patterns showing what has worked, for whom, and under what conditions. When your data resembles that of previous cases, the system infers what might help you. Statistically, this is sound reasoning. If you share genetic markers with individuals who responded well to a certain therapy, the same may hold true for you. If your biometric patterns mirror those that precede cardiac failure, a timely alert might indeed save your life.

But here lies a subtle sleight of hand. What these systems offer is not a singular understanding of you, but an inference drawn from likeness to others. It is not truly *individualised* medicine—it is refined group medicine. You are still categorised, only into smaller, more granular clusters. The algorithm doesn't know your values, your hesitations, your lived circumstances. It recognises you only insofar as you fit a pattern. And in that act of patterning, something essential—your personhood—begins to fade.

Take a concrete case: a woman in her forties learns that she carries a gene linked to heightened breast cancer risk. Predictive models recommend preventative surgery. The data, by all accounts, is accurate. Yet what the model cannot grasp is her history—her mother's trauma after undergoing the same procedure, her own uneasy relationship with medical authority, the cultural and emotional weight behind her decision to delay. The system calls her "non-compliant." She calls it "waiting." From a computational lens, she is an anomaly; from a human one, she is acting with agency and awareness.

That is not a malfunction of technology—it is a limit of its worldview.

AI excels at pattern recognition. But medicine, in its truest form, is not a science of patterns—it is the art of attending to lives. Illness unfolds not in isolation, but within biography, culture, and conscience. The human body may be quantifiable; the human experience is not. And no matter how powerful our models become, that gap—the space between pattern and person—remains stubbornly unbridgeable.

Still, the allure of algorithmic precision continues to captivate. It's not only the accuracy of AI that enchants, but the aesthetic of certainty it conveys. Dashboards shimmer with clarity, charts glide in confident symmetry, and visualisations hum with the quiet authority of numbers. These systems perform objectivity. They appear to tame the chaos of the human condition. Yet in doing so, they quietly marginalise other forms of knowledge: a clinician's intuition, a patient's narrative, even the productive ambiguity of human doubt. Where once hesitation was a mark of wisdom, it now reads as inefficiency. Where once the patient's story guided the diagnosis, it is now treated as noise to be filtered. What counts is what can be measured; what resists measurement quietly vanishes.

And so, authority begins to migrate—from person to program, from dialogue to data stream. Doctors may find themselves deferring to algorithmic recommendations that feel wrong in practice but are difficult to contest. Patients, too, can become uneasy, confronted by results that appear rational yet conflict with lived sense. The trust that once animated the clinician-patient bond shifts toward the machine, its neutrality presumed but never fully examined. Yet these systems do not operate in a vacuum. They function within institutions shaped by money, hierarchy, and habit. The appearance of objectivity masks a web of human decisions—about what constitutes evidence, what counts as compliance, and, ultimately, what counts as care.

Wearable technology illustrates this tension vividly. These sleek devices promise to know our bodies in real time—tracking pulse, glucose, sleep, even mood—feeding insights to apps that tell us how healthy, productive, or "balanced" we are. It is, undeniably, a feat of engineering. Yet it quietly reframes our relationship with ourselves. Health becomes a dashboard metric; wellbeing, a performance index. The more we gaze at these metrics, the more our sense of normality is defined by their readouts. Any deviation becomes a problem to be corrected, no matter how benign.

That redefinition carries a cost. As personalisation collapses into quantification, ordinary human variation risks being pathologised. The person with restless sleep is nudged toward "improvement" they may neither want nor need. The adolescent flagged for "elevated anxiety" by passive monitoring might find themselves medicalised before they have even named their feelings. Beneath it all lies a presumption that data knows best—that health is an objective constant, deviation a defect.

But that presumption is not purely technical—it is cultural. The faith in data stems not only from what machines can achieve, but from what we wish they could guarantee. We crave clarity amidst uncertainty, efficiency amidst chaos, certainty amidst care. We want to believe that technology can spare us the unease of ambiguity. And so, we lend it a moral authority it neither claims nor deserves.

The real challenge, then, is not merely to expose the limits of AI, but to interrogate our own readiness to believe in its myths. Personalisation, as currently practised, is no neutral progress—it is an ideology shaped by profit, by power, by a culture enamoured with control. It substitutes correlation for conversation, context for calculation. It promises to know us, but often erases the very aspects that make us knowable to one another.

In the pages ahead, we will peel back this illusion. We will examine the rise of personalised medicine, the workings of predictive modelling, and the uneasy coexistence of algorithmic insight and clinical wisdom. We will ask not only what data reveals, but what it conceals. And we will search for a vision of personalisation that restores what has quietly been lost: narrative, meaning, choice.

The task is not to reject precision, but to see beyond it—to recognise its truths without mistaking them for the whole truth. Only then can we begin to imagine a medicine that is both technologically advanced and, in the deepest sense, humane.

The Promise of Tailored Medicine

The notion that medicine could one day be uniquely suited to each individual has long occupied the imagination of clinicians, researchers, and patients alike. It appeals not only to scientific curiosity, but to a deeply personal desire: the wish to be seen, known, and treated as a singular being rather than as an anonymous body within a diagnostic category. Today, artificial intelligence offers to fulfil that wish—not as aspiration, but as application. Through the convergence of genomics, real-time biometric tracking, and predictive analytics, healthcare is entering what is widely heralded as a new age of hyper-personalisation. The claim is not modest. It is, in many cases, nothing short of transformational: algorithms that promise to detect illness before it manifests, tailor treatments down to the molecular level, and monitor physiology with such granularity that care becomes anticipatory rather than reactive.

At the heart of this vision is a powerful message: that individuality is not an obstacle to medical progress, but its new foundation. Unlike the medicine of the past—formulated on the basis of population-level averages and generalised pathways—AI-driven personalisation proposes a future in which treatment is sculpted precisely to the contours of one's genetic, behavioural, and environmental data. The "right drug, for the right person, at the right time" is no longer a slogan of medical idealism; it is increasingly positioned as a technological certainty.

And yet, the closer one examines this promise, the more complex and conditional it becomes.

Personalised medicine, as it is currently marketed, rests on a conflation between two very different ideas: *specificity* and *individuality*. Specificity refers to the capacity of technology to operate at ever finer levels of detail—identifying a mutation, tracking a biomarker, predicting a risk. Individuality, however, concerns the lived reality of a person—how they experience illness, how they make decisions, and how they locate meaning in their health. The promise of tailored medicine hinges on the assumption that the former reliably captures the latter. It assumes that because our biology can now be modelled more precisely, our care has become more personal. But this is a profound leap, and not an uncontested one.

To understand the nature of this leap, it helps to begin with genomics—the flagship domain of personalised medicine. In recent years, the cost of sequencing the human genome has fallen precipitously, enabling a growing number of individuals to have their DNA analysed for susceptibility to disease, pharmacological compatibility, and even lifestyle recommendations. The hope is clear: that by understanding the genetic underpinnings of health and disease, we can deliver interventions that are not merely targeted, but optimised for the individual.

In oncology, for instance, genomic sequencing has enabled the rise of "precision therapies" that target the molecular drivers of specific tumours. In pharmacogenomics, patients can be screened to determine which medications are likely to be effective or cause adverse effects, reducing trial-and-error prescribing. These are genuine breakthroughs, and they offer a glimpse of a future in which medicine is more responsive to biological variation.

But they also illuminate the limits of that responsiveness. For one, genetic data is inherently probabilistic. It may indicate a higher or lower risk for certain conditions, but it does not determine their inevitability. Lifestyle, environment, epigenetic factors, and socio-economic context all play a role—factors that lie largely outside the purview of genetic modelling. Furthermore, the vast majority of genomic studies have been conducted on populations of European ancestry, raising urgent questions about the applicability of their findings to global populations. What is "personalised" in one context may be partial or misleading in another.

Then there is the question of how predictive analytics translates into practice. Increasingly, machine learning models are trained on electronic health records, clinical imaging, lab results, and even patient-reported outcomes to generate risk scores and treatment recommendations. In intensive care units, AI systems flag early signs of deterioration. In primary care, decision-support tools suggest potential diagnoses based on symptom clusters. In mental health, apps track language patterns or social media behaviour to detect depressive trends.

These systems are sophisticated, but they are not omniscient. Their effectiveness is bounded by the data on which they are trained, and by the assumptions encoded into their design. They work well in environments where patterns are stable and measurable—but struggle in contexts where symptoms are diffuse, meaning is subjective, and human behaviour resists neat categorisation. A system might accurately flag a person as high-risk for cardiovascular disease based on aggregate data, but miss the fact that this person is caring for a sick parent, recently lost a job, or is dealing with chronic stress—all factors that shape both the expression of illness and the appropriateness of care.

The same principle applies to wearable technologies, which now occupy a central role in the personalisation narrative. Devices such as smartwatches, glucose monitors, and sleep trackers generate continuous streams of data that feed into health dashboards and behaviour-modification tools. These devices claim to offer insights into one's health status, often using gamification or nudges to encourage lifestyle adjustments. In theory, they empower the user to become an active participant in their own care.

In practice, however, the relationship between data and agency is more ambiguous. The information produced by wearables is only as meaningful as the framework through which it is interpreted. High heart rate variability may be a sign of fitness in one context, or anxiety in another. Poor sleep quality may reflect a physiological problem, or simply a misalignment between tracking algorithms and lived experience. Moreover, the very act of quantifying health can shift the user's relationship to their body—from intuitive awareness to analytical scrutiny. What was once felt is now measured; what was once lived is now logged.

This shift is not without consequence. It introduces a new layer of self-surveillance into everyday life, where deviations from algorithmic norms trigger alerts, recommendations, or feelings of failure. The user may come to trust the device more than their own perception—accepting the authority of the data even when it contradicts experience. This is not empowerment; it is a subtle form of dependency, and one that recasts health not as a subjective state but as a set of optimised metrics.

What ties these various applications together—genomics, predictive modelling, wearable tech—is the idea that more data will naturally yield better, more tailored care. And indeed, in many cases, it *can*. But the assumption that data equates to understanding is both philosophically and practically fragile. Knowing *what* a patient's numbers suggest is not the same as knowing *who* that patient is, or what matters to them. Data does not speak; it must be interpreted. And interpretation, especially in medicine, is never value-neutral.

This brings us to a deeper tension at the heart of AI-driven personalisation: the conflict between statistical likeness and human uniqueness. Personalised medicine operates by identifying people who resemble others in relevant ways—genetically, behaviourally, or clinically. It then applies inferences drawn from those similarities to guide treatment. This is a logical and often effective strategy. But resemblance is not identity. Two people may share a risk profile, yet diverge dramatically in how they understand, experience, or respond to illness. One may see a diagnosis as a threat; another, as a challenge. One may prioritise longevity; another, quality of life. One may accept a recommendation; another may resist it, based on prior trauma, cultural beliefs, or family obligations.

These differences are not captured in most models—not because they are unknowable, but because they are difficult to quantify. AI systems are not designed to understand meaning; they are designed to detect regularity. Their strength lies in pattern recognition, not narrative comprehension. They cannot ask a patient what they fear most about a procedure, or what their definition of a good outcome might be. They cannot detect silence, ambiguity, or ambivalence—yet these are often the most revealing elements in clinical encounters.

To treat someone based solely on their data is to risk substituting their story for a summary. And while summaries can be useful, they are never sufficient. They are maps, not terrains.

The promise of tailored medicine, then, is best understood not as a destination but as a question: *To whom, and under what conditions, does this form of care truly feel personal?* It is a question that requires constant interrogation, especially as commercial, institutional, and algorithmic forces converge to define the contours of what personalisation means. If left unchecked, we risk mistaking technical sophistication for human understanding, and in doing so, constructing a system that is personalised in theory but impersonal in practice.

The challenge is not to reject these tools, but to contextualise them. To recognise their capabilities without inflating them into fantasies. To design systems that enhance clinical insight rather than replace it. And most of all, to ensure that personalisation remains anchored in the person—not just their genes, not just their data, but their values, stories, and choices.

Medicine may be evolving rapidly, but its moral foundations remain unchanged. At its best, care is not simply about knowing more; it is about knowing wisely. Artificial intelligence may help us see more clearly—but only if we remember what we are looking *for*.

What Data Can't See

A machine learning model may correctly predict a medical emergency, but it cannot understand what it means to someone to be called "a patient." It can forecast hospital readmissions, anticipate disease progression, and infer behavioural risk factors from patterns in blood pressure, activity levels, or prescription adherence. But it cannot see a life. It cannot grasp what it is to wait six hours in a hospital corridor while caring for a child at home. It does not recognise the fatigue that accumulates not just in the body, but in the soul of someone navigating chronic illness with inadequate support. It may be impressively accurate—technically flawless—but it is, by its very nature, indifferent to context.

Lived experience is not a data point. It is dynamic, embodied, and deeply personal—woven from memory, culture, emotion, and environment. It emerges through time, conversation, and vulnerability. And yet, in the data-first paradigm of AI-driven healthcare, this is the element that disappears. The focus narrows to what can be measured, modelled, and predicted. What cannot be rendered into a variable is treated, at best, as anecdotal. At worst, it is ignored entirely.

The consequences of this omission are rarely theoretical. Consider a real case from a large North American health system where a predictive model was used to identify patients at high risk of hospital readmission. The algorithm, built on a dataset of insurance claims and clinical records, accurately stratified patients based on prior healthcare utilisation. One patient—a 74-year-old woman with multiple chronic conditions—was flagged as low-risk. She had few hospital visits on record and appeared stable. Yet within weeks, she was re-admitted in crisis. What the model couldn't see was her housing instability, her isolation after the death of her spouse, and her reluctance to seek care because of prior discrimination. These weren't captured in billing data or clinical summaries. But they shaped her health far more powerfully than any lab value.

This is not an isolated failure. Numerous studies have revealed how data-driven tools misclassify or overlook individuals whose health profiles deviate from statistical norms—not due to physiological differences, but because their lives unfold in contexts the system has not been trained to recognise. AI may infer that a person is non-compliant with medication because they haven't filled a prescription. It cannot see that the pharmacy is two bus rides away, or that the person prioritised food over medication in a week of impossible choices.

There is a growing body of evidence to suggest that these models often perform worst for those who are already underserved: racial minorities, individuals with disabilities, people living in poverty, and those whose interactions with the healthcare system have been shaped by stigma, mistrust, or trauma. The issue is not simply one of biased data—though that is part of it—it is that *experience itself* has been excluded from the ontology of the model. The model does not fail because it is malicious. It fails because it was never taught to look for what matters.

What this reveals is a deeper epistemological problem. In the world of machine learning, knowledge is derived from correlation. Meaning emerges from the repetition of patterns across large datasets. But human health is not simply a pattern to be recognised. It is also a story to be told. Diagnosis, treatment, and recovery are not just biological events—they are lived narratives, often shaped by fear, agency, shame, and meaning. When we reduce the patient to a cluster of metrics, we do not merely oversimplify—we actively distort.

Take, for example, the use of natural language processing to analyse physician notes. These systems are designed to detect key terms and extract structured data from free-text documentation. They are efficient, scalable, and, in many cases, highly effective at identifying mentions of conditions, symptoms, or interventions. But they miss tone. They miss irony. They miss the subtext of a physician documenting that a patient is "doing fine," while knowing full well that the phrase masks deterioration softened for the family. They miss the tension in a note dictated after a difficult conversation, or the clinical restraint used when describing a patient whose decisions the clinician does not support. No matter how advanced the algorithm, it cannot interpret silence.

This limitation becomes even more visible in mental health care, where lived experience is not ancillary but central. A chatbot may screen for depression based on user responses. A sentiment analysis model may track changes in tone or language over time. But they cannot parse the layered meaning of ambivalence, the cultural nuances of how distress is communicated, or the protective silences people maintain when they sense they are not safe to speak freely. In these cases, accuracy is not enough. What matters is *attunement*—and that remains the province of human attention.

The allure of machine learning is its promise to make sense of complexity at scale. But the type of sense it makes is statistical, not situated. It is a kind of knowledge that privileges abstraction over specificity. A risk score may correctly rank a population, but offer little insight into any one person's experience. This is not a flaw in design—it is a feature of the paradigm. Machine learning excels when the goal is to generalise. But medicine, at its best, is relational. It listens before it calculates. It considers what matters to the person, not just what is likely to happen.

What makes this tension more acute is the rhetoric surrounding AI. Terms like "objective," "evidence-based," and "data-driven" carry the aura of authority. They suggest that human fallibility is being corrected, that care is finally being liberated from bias and intuition. But this is a dangerous illusion. The data itself is not neutral. It reflects the history, structure, and blind spots of the systems that produced it. If certain populations have worse documented outcomes, the model may interpret this as a characteristic of those patients rather than an indictment of the care they received. If pain scores are consistently underreported in women or people of colour, the model will learn that they are less likely to be in pain.

Lived experience resists formalisation. It resists the neat boundaries of datasets and the structured inputs that machine learning requires. But it is precisely this messiness that makes it essential. Illness is not merely a deviation from the biological norm—it is a rupture in a life. It disrupts plans, identity, relationships. It calls into question one's sense of control, belonging, and hope. These dimensions do not appear in lab results or diagnostic codes. But they shape whether a patient will follow through with treatment, whether they will trust a clinician, and whether they will feel cared for.

The temptation, in systems engineering, is to treat these elements as externalities—as "soft" variables that lie outside the remit of computational modelling. But to do so is to misunderstand the practice of medicine. A doctor who misses a diagnosis because of a rare presentation has made a technical error. But a doctor who fails to hear what the diagnosis means to the patient has failed in a more profound way. AI, in its current form, cannot correct for this. It can assist. It can alert. It can refine. But it cannot *care*.

To build systems that serve rather than obscure the human dimensions of health, we must shift our orientation. Rather than asking how to extract more data from the patient, we must ask how to preserve the patient's voice within the system. This means designing models that are not only accurate, but interpretable. It means integrating narrative forms of documentation—not to be reduced to sentiment scores, but to be *read*. It means involving patients in the design of technologies that affect them, ensuring that the questions asked by machines are grounded in the concerns of those who live with the answers.

Most importantly, it means recognising that the greatest insights often emerge not from what the data shows, but from what it omits. The story that was never documented. The symptom that was dismissed. The patient who didn't return.

What data can't see is not irrelevant. It is precisely where meaning resides. And until we make room for that meaning—within our models, our metrics, and our mindsets—we will continue to mistake prediction for understanding. We will continue to build systems that are technically correct, and yet profoundly disconnected from the people they aim to serve.

Personhood vs. Pattern Recognition

A machine can detect the subtle radiographic signs of pneumonia long before a human eye would register the anomaly. It can estimate cardiovascular risk more accurately than many physicians, given the right data. It can scan millions of health records in seconds, infer relationships, and generate probabilistic insights with astonishing efficiency. What it cannot do—and perhaps never will—is ask, *Why now?* Why did this patient, with this condition, come forward at this moment? What emotional threshold was crossed, what conversation finally gave them permission to acknowledge their pain? The answer lies not in pattern, but in personhood.

The central tension facing modern medicine is no longer merely between art and science, or between clinical discretion and protocol. It is between *recognition of pattern* and *recognition of self.* Artificial intelligence systems operate on the premise that health, illness, and behaviour can be reduced to statistically significant signatures—patterns waiting to be discerned in genomic sequences, sensor data, or patient histories. But care—real care—demands more than recognition of recurrence. It demands *acknowledgment of uniqueness*, of subjectivity, of meaning. And meaning, as every experienced clinician knows, often lives in the places machines cannot reach.

Consider the following scenario. A 52-year-old man presents at an emergency department with chest pain. An AI triage system—trained on thousands of cases—assesses his electrocardiogram, cross-references it with vital signs, previous admissions, and lab values, and assigns him a low probability of myocardial infarction. The physician, reading the same data, hesitates. Something about the man's presentation, his guarded manner, his comment that "this feels different," triggers concern. She overrides the triage algorithm, admits him for observation, and hours later, the patient deteriorates rapidly. A major coronary event is confirmed.

Was the algorithm wrong? Not in its own terms. Statistically, it made a reasonable prediction based on the information available. But it missed what the physician caught: *subtext, pattern disrupted by context*, the *discrepancy between what is said and what is meant*. It is in this space—between statistical pattern and human story—that medical judgment lives. And it is precisely this space that algorithmic models struggle to occupy.

Medical intuition is often caricatured as unscientific or unreliable—a residue of pre-digital practice. But this is a mischaracterisation. Intuition in medicine is not guesswork; it is pattern recognition enriched by *relational memory, ethical attunement*, and *narrative competence*. It draws on thousands of prior encounters, but also on the clinician's awareness of the person in front of them—their tone, affect, hesitations, the broader arc of their life. It is reasoning, yes, but reasoning that is *embodied, contextual*, and often *inarticulable*. You know something is wrong because something *feels* wrong—and that feeling emerges not from superstition, but from a sophisticated, if often subconscious, calibration of cues.

Algorithmic prediction, by contrast, is formal, explicit, and reproducible. It does not feel. It calculates. Its strength lies in consistency, scalability, and the ability to detect patterns invisible to the human eye. It is not undermined by fatigue, mood, or bias in the moment of decision. But it is also *impervious to meaning*. A model may note that a patient is at high risk for treatment non-adherence, based on historical data. It cannot know that the patient is newly motivated by the birth of a grandchild, or that they recently joined a community support group. It may see recidivism where there is now resolve.

This creates a new kind of dissonance in clinical practice. Doctors are increasingly being asked to reconcile their subjective impressions with objective outputs. When the two align, confidence is bolstered. But when they conflict, tension emerges. Should the clinician defer to the model, knowing its recommendations are grounded in far more data than any individual could process? Or should they trust their intuition, even when the algorithm disagrees?

These are not theoretical dilemmas. In hospitals across the world, clinicians face such choices daily—decisions that require navigating the complex terrain between *probability* and *possibility*, *efficiency* and *empathy*. A paediatrician treating a non-verbal autistic child may override a digital triage suggestion, sensing distress that the system cannot register. A palliative care physician may resist a predictive mortality score, recognising that the patient is not ready to confront such prognostication. In these moments, the clinician is not rejecting science—they are invoking *judgement*, informed by science but accountable to the person.

What makes this dynamic more fraught is the institutional context in which it unfolds. Many healthcare systems, under pressure to optimise resources, now embed AI into their core operations—not as tools to assist, but as structures to govern. Algorithmic outputs shape referrals, determine eligibility for services, and flag "at-risk" patients for targeted interventions. The language used is one of *support*, but the function is often one of *control*. When an algorithm flags a patient as low priority, the burden shifts to the clinician to justify deviation. When a model recommends a course of action, resistance can be seen as inefficiency—or even liability.

In this environment, the space for clinical judgement shrinks. The clinician becomes a manager of risk rather than a steward of care. The patient becomes a site of optimisation rather than a subject of interpretation. This is not a hypothetical dystopia—it is a quietly encroaching reality, enabled not by coercion, but by the rhetoric of objectivity. The more we frame algorithms as neutral, the more we sideline those aspects of care that are inherently *interpretive*, *ethical*, and *relational*.

To defend the importance of personhood in medicine is not to romanticise the past, nor to reject the real benefits of AI. It is to assert that *understanding* is not reducible to *prediction*. That even perfect foresight offers no substitute for *presence*. That knowing what is likely to happen is not the same as knowing *what matters most* if it does.

This distinction becomes especially vital in fields where care involves not just diagnosis and treatment, but *witnessing*, *accompaniment*, and *meaning-making*. In mental health, oncology, geriatrics, and palliative care, the role of the clinician extends beyond clinical intervention to include the navigation of existential questions: *How do I live with this condition? What am I willing to endure? What does healing mean for me now?* These are not questions a model can answer. They require conversation, listening, and the courage to hold uncertainty.

There is, of course, a place for pattern recognition in all of this. No physician can see every possibility. No human can recall every permutation of symptoms. AI can extend our vision—but only if we remain the ones who decide where to look, and why. The danger lies not in using algorithms, but in forgetting their limits. In mistaking a well-fitted model for a full picture. In allowing statistical insight to become a substitute for relational engagement.

True personalisation in medicine does not begin with a dataset. It begins with a question, asked in real time, of a real person, in a room where presence still matters: *What brings you here today?* Not just what hurts, but what else is happening. Not just what we can treat, but what the patient is hoping for. No model, however sophisticated, can ask that question meaningfully. No algorithm can hear the silence that sometimes follows.

The future of care will almost certainly include machines that are faster, smarter, and more "objective" than the clinicians who use them. But whether that future serves patients as persons—or merely optimises their care as patterns—depends on whether we preserve the space for judgment that only humans can occupy. Not because machines are incapable, but because *we* are responsible.

That responsibility includes knowing when to trust the model—and when to trust the story. When to lean on data—and when to lean in. When the prediction makes sense—and when the person reminds us why it doesn't. Only then can we honour both the science of medicine and the humanity it is meant to serve.

The Algorithmic Aesthetic

A beautifully rendered interface can make a lie feel like truth. In healthcare, where stakes are existential and decisions intimate, this matters more than we often admit. The appeal of AI-powered medicine is not merely technical—it is aesthetic. Precision, in this context, is not just a claim about accuracy; it is a *look*, a *feel*, a *promise* of order imposed upon biological and human complexity. It speaks in the visual language of clean lines, sharp typography, seamless dashboards, and glowing status bars—each element carefully constructed to evoke mastery, efficiency, and calm. But what is often overlooked is that this aesthetic, while reassuring, can also obscure the limits of what such systems truly understand.

We are conditioned to trust the appearance of control. A diagnostic tool that displays risk scores in red, amber, or green feels more trustworthy than a clinician expressing uncertainty. A decision support system that presents a treatment pathway through a crisp interface seems more rational than a doctor who hesitates, asks more questions, and weighs possibilities aloud. The former conveys resolution. The latter signals complexity. In a culture that values speed, productivity, and clarity, complexity becomes uncomfortable—even suspect. The algorithmic aesthetic exploits this discomfort, offering answers with the kind of assurance that human cognition rarely delivers without caveats.

This aesthetic is not incidental. It is engineered. Tech companies invest heavily in user experience (UX) design to ensure that their platforms *feel* intuitive, authoritative, and modern. In healthcare, these visual and interactional cues do more than streamline workflows—they encode an entire epistemology. The interface becomes the message. And when an AI tool is wrapped in the design conventions of Silicon Valley minimalism—white space, neutral tones, dynamic infographics—it inherits a set of cultural assumptions: that it is objective, future-facing, and unburdened by human error. The messiness of medicine—the contradictions, the tensions, the doubts—disappears behind a frictionless UI.

This frictionlessness is seductive because it matches a broader cultural moment. In an age saturated with data and paralysed by decision fatigue, the appeal of a tool that simplifies the world into actionable metrics is powerful. It mirrors the apps we use to navigate, to sleep, to parent, to optimise our productivity. In this sense, the algorithmic aesthetic in healthcare is not just a design choice—it is a manifestation of a worldview. One that prizes clarity over ambiguity, logic over empathy, and predictability over presence.

Yet medicine is not, and has never been, reducible to input-output functions. The human body may follow biological laws, but illness unfolds within social, emotional, and cultural contexts. A system may report that a patient's vital signs are within range, but it cannot know that they are experiencing grief that will manifest as fatigue and low appetite. A model may generate a treatment recommendation based on population-level data, but it cannot sense the discomfort in a patient's eyes as they imagine the implications of that treatment for their work, their relationships, their sense of self.

These are not marginal concerns. They are central to care. And when systems present themselves with the polished confidence of total comprehension, they make it harder for both patients and clinicians to question them. The veneer of precision becomes a form of epistemic authority—implied, not argued. Doubt becomes irrational. Deviation becomes inefficiency.

The cultural appeal of precision is deeply historical. Since the Enlightenment, medicine has drawn legitimacy from its alignment with scientific rationalism. The shift from humoral theory to cellular pathology, from bedside to bench, from case history to laboratory test—all have reinforced the image of medicine as a discipline grounded in measurable fact. AI extends this tradition, but with a crucial difference: its tools do not always offer interpretability. A clinician might understand the mechanism behind a stethoscope or an MRI. But the internal logic of a neural network, trained on millions of data points, remains opaque even to its creators. What is offered in place of explanation is visual elegance—high-resolution dashboards, precise percentages, neat correlations.

This replacement of interpretability with aesthetics introduces a new form of risk: *overtrust*. Studies have shown that clinicians are more likely to accept algorithmic outputs that are presented in polished formats, even when they contradict clinical intuition. This effect is amplified in time-pressured environments, where decision fatigue and institutional protocols create strong incentives to defer to the system. Patients, too, are influenced by design. A health app that visualises sleep stages with animated charts appears more accurate than one that displays raw data—even if both are based on the same flawed assumptions about what sleep metrics can capture.

The problem is not that these systems are useless. Many offer real benefits: faster triage, early detection, workload reduction. The issue is that their aesthetic often exceeds their epistemic warrant. They *look* like they understand more than they do. And this appearance shapes behaviour.

A striking example can be found in oncology, where decision-support systems increasingly offer personalised treatment plans based on genetic profiling and outcomes data. These tools often present recommendations alongside confidence intervals, peer-reviewed references, and ranking scores—all rendered through elegant interfaces. But the complexity behind these outputs—differing trial designs, population biases, contextual limitations—is largely invisible. The design implies neutrality. The system becomes the authority. And in doing so, it shifts the locus of trust from the clinician-patient relationship to the machine.

This shift is not neutral. It reflects broader trends in technoculture: the elevation of optimisation as a moral good, the framing of uncertainty as a problem to be solved algorithmically, and the transformation of human variation into a design problem. When applied to medicine, these values can displace more humanistic forms of knowledge—story, narrative, ethical discernment—with forms that are quantifiable, traceable, and auditable. What can be rendered as a variable is privileged. What cannot be measured is marginalised.

This has implications not only for individual care, but for institutional governance. As hospitals and health systems adopt AI tools at scale, metrics and interfaces begin to shape how success is defined. Clinical pathways are standardised not only through evidence, but through what is legible to the algorithm. "Personalised care" becomes what the system can calculate, not what the patient articulates. Risk scores, rather than narrative nuance, determine resource allocation. And in the background, the aesthetic of the system continues to reassure all involved that progress is being made.

To resist this drift, it is not enough to design more "transparent" AI. Transparency, while important, does not fully address the seductions of form. A well-annotated model can still present misleading confidence if wrapped in an interface that signals authority. Nor is the solution to abandon design altogether. *Good design matters*—it enables accessibility, reduces cognitive load, and improves usability. But it must be *honest design*. Design that signals its limitations as clearly as its capacities. That invites questions rather than silencing them. That foregrounds interpretation over automation.

This requires a shift in how we educate both clinicians and patients. Visual literacy must become part of clinical training—not just in reading radiographs, but in critically assessing the design choices that shape AI interfaces. Patients, too, must be supported to interpret the tools they use, not merely comply with their recommendations. And developers must be accountable not only for the accuracy of their models, but for the epistemological claims their designs imply.

What is ultimately at stake in the algorithmic aesthetic is not just a question of style, but of *truth*. Not truth in the sense of technical correctness, but in the sense of care that is honest about what it knows and what it does not. The systems we build reflect the values we encode. If we prioritise polish over humility, certainty over curiosity, prediction over presence, we will get systems that are efficient but blind.

Precision, properly understood, is not the elimination of ambiguity. It is the disciplined confrontation of it. And that is a task no design, however elegant, can do on its own. It must be embedded in a practice of care that remembers that the appearance of understanding is not the same as understanding itself. That the map is not the territory. And that the cleanest interface can sometimes conceal the deepest silence.

Chapter 2
From Diagnosis to Datafication

Before a patient is reduced to a chart, they are a body. And before that chart becomes a dataset, it is a story—told in gestures, symptoms, hesitations, and quiet exchanges. Medicine was born in that very space: the interpretive encounter between one person seeking help and another striving to understand. Today, that space is shrinking. It is being colonised by a new order of knowledge—one that privileges data over dialogue, quantification over meaning. What once began as an act of interpretation has been reconstituted as an act of computation. The human body, once read as narrative, is now parsed as information.

This is more than a technical adjustment. It represents a philosophical and institutional upheaval. In its pursuit of precision, modern medicine has reimagined illness as information, and care as calculation. Blood pressure becomes a graph, mood becomes a metric, movement dissolves into gait analysis, and risk appears as a heatmap. These are all rendered legible to systems that cannot comprehend suffering or hope but are masters of inference. The subjective realm of illness—the lived, felt, often messy part of being unwell—has not vanished; it has merely been demoted, relegated beneath whatever can be digitised and fed into a model.

This did not happen in a single technological leap. The quantification of the body has been centuries in the making. Its intellectual roots reach back to the Enlightenment, when medicine began its long separation from philosophy and theology, seeking the clarity of science. The invention of the stethoscope in 1816 marked a turning point—not just in practice but in perception. For the first time, physicians could listen directly to the inner workings of the body. A patient's narrative gave way to a pulse of sound; the story became a signal. Thermometers, sphygmomanometers, ECGs—each extended human perception while subtly redefining what counted as knowledge. The medical gaze, as Foucault put it, turned inward—towards the measurable, the anatomical, the empirically legible.

And yet, those early instruments still required interpretation. They were tools in the hands of practitioners schooled not only in physiology but in judgment. Diagnosis was an evolving conversation, a negotiation between observation and intuition. The doctor listened—not only with the ear or the eye, but with the imagination. Evidence was gathered, yes, but meaning was made.

Today, the shift is not simply in the use of data, but in its dominion. We inhabit an era in which data no longer supports medical judgment—it supplants it. Clinical reasoning is increasingly mediated by decision-support systems trained on vast archives of patient information. These machine learning models are built to predict, not to explain. They are judged by their accuracy, not their coherence. Their inner workings—dense with nonlinear correlations—are largely opaque even to those who deploy them. We have, in effect, exchanged interpretability for performance.

The implications of that exchange are not theoretical. Take, for instance, a hospital that employs an algorithm to forecast sepsis risk. It sifts through thousands of data points—vitals, lab results, medication history—and issues a score. If the score crosses a threshold, an alert triggers early intervention. On paper, this saves lives. But for the clinician, the number arrives without narrative. The model cannot explain its conclusion in the language of human reasoning—it cannot say, "The patient's pressure has dipped, their white count is climbing, their lactate is creeping up." It merely pronounces:

high risk. Trusting such a judgment becomes, oddly, a matter of faith.

This dependence on "black box" systems subtly recasts the physician's role. The doctor becomes an interpreter of predictions they did not derive, a custodian of accountability for decisions they only partially authored. They must reconcile machine authority with human responsibility—a tension that medicine is not well equipped to resolve. How does one justify a decision that one cannot fully explain? Where, in such a hybrid logic, does moral agency reside?

This tension plays out daily, often invisibly. And it deepens when we confront the biases that are built into the data itself. Machine learning does not operate on truth; it operates on history. It sees patterns in what has already happened. If that history is unjust, the injustice becomes algorithmic. Suppose a dataset reflects that Black patients historically received less pain medication than white patients. The model may infer, quite "rationally," that Black patients experience or report less pain. What it learns, in other words, is discrimination rendered as data.

The results can be quietly catastrophic. In one prominent case, a commercial risk tool used in American hospitals consistently underestimated the needs of Black patients. Its designers had used healthcare spending as a proxy for health status—assuming that sicker patients cost more to treat. But because systemic inequities limit access to care, Black patients appeared, on paper, healthier than they truly were. The algorithm was not malicious; it was merely obedient. It replicated the bias it inherited.

Here lies a hard truth: data is never neutral. It bears the imprint of the institutions, incentives, and omissions that created it. It reflects who is recorded, how, and for what purpose. Once these traces become the scaffolding for predictive models, their distortions harden into policy. Bias ceases to be a historical footnote and becomes operational fact.

Consider now a case where the system performed exactly as intended—and still failed. A woman in her thirties arrives at a clinic complaining of vague abdominal pain. Her vital signs are stable, her bloodwork unremarkable. The AI model, trained on millions of prior cases, calculates a low probability of appendicitis. The clinician, pressed for time, accepts the model's reassurance and sends her home. Hours later, her appendix ruptures.

Statistically, the model was correct: the vast majority of similar patients did not have appendicitis. But statistics deal in likelihoods, not lives. The model could not perceive the small cues—the guarded movement, the unease that defies metrics, the intuition that something is amiss. Those are not data points. They are forms of knowing that no algorithm can yet grasp.

The lesson is stark: care is always particular. Models reason across populations; medicine acts on individuals. Predictions describe trends, but illness resists abstraction. When a model's forecast is mistaken for fact, the clinician's interpretive role shrinks, and the patient's voice risks becoming irrelevant. Medicine turns from conversation to compliance.

This chapter unpacks that transformation—the drift from diagnosis as interpretation to diagnosis as computation. It follows the historical, philosophical, and technical pathways that brought us here. It examines how AI systems both enhance and constrain medical judgment, offering speed and scale but stripping away transparency. It explores how bias seeps into code, how algorithms perpetuate inequality under the guise of objectivity, and how a statistically flawless model can still betray the singular patient before it.

The argument is not anti-technology. It is, rather, a plea for lucidity. Predictive accuracy is not understanding. Optimisation is not justice. And when the human body becomes a dataset, something of its mystery—its dignity—is put at risk. To preserve that humanity, we do not need less data. We need deeper reflection on how, and why, we choose to trust it.

How the Body Became a Dataset

If you ask a physician today what it means to "know" a patient, the answer will almost certainly begin with data. Vital signs, lab values, genetic profiles, imaging results, electronic health records—the modern patient is presented less as a person and more as a structured accumulation of numbers, categories, and codes. Their story, once central to the clinical encounter, is now bracketed by standardised templates and algorithmic inferences. A diagnosis no longer emerges through dialogue alone; it is increasingly derived from correlations, extracted from datasets, and evaluated against probabilistic thresholds. What has changed is not merely the technology of medicine, but its epistemology. *Care is no longer simply interpreted—it is computed.*

This shift, profound though it is, did not begin with machine learning or wearable sensors. The quantification of the body has a long and deliberate history—rooted not in malice or mechanisation, but in a drive for accuracy, consistency, and control. For centuries, physicians relied heavily on narrative accounts and subjective impressions. Illness was described, not measured. Symptoms were contextualised through culture, memory, and metaphor. But as medicine aligned itself with the scientific method during the Enlightenment, it began to distance itself from ambiguity. Observation gave way to instrumentation. Personal testimony yielded to objective metrics. The body became not just something to listen to, but something to read—and eventually, to calculate.

The 19th century marked a turning point. With the introduction of tools like the stethoscope (1816), the thermometer (mid-1800s), and the sphygmomanometer (1881), clinicians were now able to access the body's internal states without relying solely on a patient's words. These instruments did more than improve diagnosis; they shifted the locus of clinical authority. What mattered was not how illness felt, but what it measured. Pain could be localised, temperature indexed, pulse recorded. The subjective began to lose ground to the standardised.

This evolution accelerated in the 20th century with the rise of biomedicine and hospital-based care. Laboratory testing, imaging technologies, and electronic health records all contributed to the fragmentation of the body into traceable, storable elements. Blood glucose levels, oxygen saturation, creatinine clearance—each offered a data point to be monitored, trended, and optimised. The goal was clear: to reduce uncertainty. But the trade-off was less frequently acknowledged. As measurement expanded, so too did a quiet redefinition of what it meant to be *seen* by medicine. The patient became legible insofar as they were quantifiable.

The philosophical implications of this shift are not incidental. When medicine was primarily interpretive, it required engagement with narrative, with complexity, and with meaning. A diagnosis was not only a label, but an act of discernment—a hypothesis that needed to account for lived experience. A clinician had to consider not just *what* was wrong, but *why now, in this person, in this life*. But as diagnostic tools became more powerful and more abstract, that interpretive stance gave way to a computational one. The clinician ceased to be an interpreter of illness and became a navigator of systems. And the patient was no longer someone whose story needed to be heard, but someone whose data needed to be entered, processed, and scored.

This reorientation is now reaching its most intensified form through AI-powered systems that operate entirely within the realm of data. Predictive analytics does not require a story. It requires enough past examples to infer patterns. The value of a patient is not in their uniqueness, but in their similarity to others who have come before. Risk is not a matter of clinical gestalt—it is a percentile. Diagnosis is not a judgment—it is a probability. And the body is not a subject—it is a statistical entity.

Biometric monitoring completes the transformation. Wearables, smartphone sensors, implantables—all function to generate continuous streams of data, parsing the body in real time. These devices are marketed not simply as conveniences, but as instruments of empowerment. The user, we are told, becomes their own diagnostician. Health becomes a series of dashboards. Deviations from algorithmically defined norms are flagged, nudged, and sometimes medicalised. But what's often overlooked is that these systems do not merely report—they *define* what counts as health, risk, or normalcy. The ontology of the body is being written in code, shaped by design choices, business models, and assumptions that are rarely transparent to the user.

The shift from care as interpretation to care as computation is not inherently malign. It has delivered undeniable advances: early detection of disease, improved consistency in decision-making, reductions in human error. But it also raises profound questions. What happens to the experience of illness when it is mediated entirely through metrics? What is lost when the clinician relies on algorithmic outputs instead of listening to the patient's account? How do we navigate a system that increasingly equates health with data integrity?

The clinical consequences of this shift are now coming into sharp focus. Consider the patient whose blood pressure appears stable on the monitor, but who is visibly pale and short of breath. Or the older adult whose biometric indicators fall within normal ranges, but whose weight loss, apathy, and confusion suggest something more insidious. In these cases, the numbers do not lie—but they also do not speak the whole truth. The data is accurate, but incomplete. And without interpretive attention, the risk is not miscalculation—it is *misunderstanding*.

There is also a cognitive toll on clinicians. As diagnostic reasoning becomes increasingly data-dependent, the role of the physician shifts from detective to adjudicator. Instead of asking, "What is the underlying cause of this presentation?", they are asked to evaluate whether a model's prediction is worth overruling. The epistemic authority of the doctor is diluted—not by evidence, but by automation. Trust becomes procedural rather than relational. And when errors occur, they are harder to trace: was it the data, the model, the interface, or the decision-maker?

One might argue that the problem is not with data, but with its use. This is only partly true. *How* data is used matters. But so does *what* is considered data in the first place. Most AI systems treat the body as a collection of signals—heart rate variability, gait analysis, oxygen saturation, voice cadence. But they struggle with what philosopher Annemarie Mol calls "the logic of care"—the messy, negotiated, context-dependent nature of what it means to live with illness. A patient might "fail" to adhere to a medication schedule, not because of ignorance, but because they prioritise caring for a parent. They might "deviate" from a treatment plan because of spiritual beliefs. These are not errors in logic. They are expressions of life. But to a system optimised for compliance and pattern recognition, they appear as anomalies to be corrected.

This discrepancy is not just theoretical—it has policy implications. Insurance companies increasingly use predictive analytics to assess risk and allocate resources. Employers monitor employee wellness through biometric platforms. Public health agencies use aggregated data to shape interventions. In each case, the body becomes a data source, and the person a node in a risk matrix. The human dimensions of illness—grief, uncertainty, hope—are flattened into variables. And once something is measured, it is subject to control. What begins as care can quickly drift toward surveillance.

To respond to this reality, we must reassert a crucial distinction: data is not the body. It is a translation. And like all translations, it involves selection, omission, and interpretation. The dataset is not a mirror of the person—it is a construct, shaped by what was collected, how it was coded, and what was deemed relevant. This does not make it useless. But it does make it partial. And when we forget that, we risk mistaking abstraction for presence.

The future of medicine will almost certainly involve more data, not less. But the challenge is to ensure that this data serves the practice of care, rather than replacing it. That it enriches human judgment, rather than displacing it. That it supports the complexity of illness, rather than collapsing it into a series of metrics. This is not a call to nostalgia. It is a call to clarity. The body did not become a dataset by accident. It became one through choices—historical, institutional, technical. Those choices can be re-examined. And new ones can be made. Choices that remember that medicine is not just about managing information. It is about understanding lives.

Clinical Judgment in the Age of Black Boxes

In medicine, decisions are rarely made in a vacuum. They are shaped by probabilities, but also by doubt, discretion, and the irreducible complexity of human lives. Clinical judgment—once considered the apex skill of a seasoned physician—is being recast in the shadow of algorithmic systems whose decision-making processes are powerful but increasingly inscrutable. What happens when the most authoritative tool in the room can't explain itself?

The rise of black-box models in healthcare—particularly those built using deep learning architectures—has brought with it an undeniable leap in predictive performance. Algorithms trained on hundreds of thousands of CT scans now flag early-stage cancers with greater sensitivity than many radiologists. AI systems embedded in hospital triage protocols outperform clinicians in identifying septic shock or predicting ICU admissions. The outputs are swift, impressive, and statistically robust. But they are also, more often than not, *opaque*. Even the developers of these models frequently cannot say why a particular output was generated—only that it correlates with similar past cases in a statistically significant way.

This lack of interpretability presents a sharp departure from how clinical reasoning has historically operated. A physician encountering a febrile child doesn't simply issue a binary output. They consider the history of present illness, parental concern, vital signs, prior infections, immunisation status, epidemiological trends, and the general appearance of the child—all through a combination of learned heuristics and experiential nuance. Even when uncertain, they can articulate their reasoning: "Given the duration of symptoms, lack of respiratory findings, and recent exposure to strep, I suspect a bacterial cause." The explanation may be fallible, but it is legible—open to scrutiny, debate, and modification.

Black-box AI does not function this way. It does not offer reasoning. It offers *results*. An algorithm might conclude that a patient has a 78% likelihood of readmission within 30 days, but it cannot clarify which features drove that prediction, or what underlying assumptions were embedded in its architecture. This challenges a fundamental norm of medicine: the expectation that decisions be *justifiable*. In clinical practice, justifiability is not a luxury—it is a cornerstone of trust, professional accountability, and ethical obligation.

Consider the scenario of an oncologist using a decision-support system that recommends a particular chemotherapy protocol based on molecular tumour profiling. The recommendation aligns with recent literature, but conflicts with the clinician's experience treating similar patients with comorbidities. The system cannot explain its logic beyond a citation of high-level performance metrics. Does the clinician follow the model's suggestion, potentially compromising personal judgment? Or override it, assuming the risk of going against a statistically optimised recommendation? Neither choice is straightforward—and both shift the burden of responsibility.

This tension is increasingly common. As healthcare institutions adopt AI systems across diagnostics, triage, treatment planning, and administrative oversight, clinicians are being asked to navigate a hybrid cognitive environment—one in which human reasoning must coexist with machine outputs that may be unexplainable but institutionally endorsed. And the stakes are not limited to accuracy alone. The erosion of explainability risks undermining the social fabric of medicine: the relationship between provider and patient, the ethics of informed consent, and the clinician's own sense of professional agency.

Accountability becomes slippery in such a landscape. When a decision is made based on an opaque model, and that decision leads to harm, who is responsible? The doctor who accepted the recommendation? The institution that purchased the system? The vendor who trained the model on a proprietary dataset? The very structure of clinical accountability—rooted in the ability to trace and evaluate the reasoning behind decisions—is strained under the weight of systems that produce results without rationale.

To be clear, the opacity of these systems is not the result of careless design. It is an intrinsic feature of certain machine learning approaches. Deep neural networks, for instance, derive their predictive power from the layered processing of vast amounts of input data—often involving millions of parameters and nonlinear transformations. These architectures were not built to explain their conclusions in human terms; they were built to optimise outcomes. But in the domain of medicine, where transparency and trust are interdependent, this optimisation is not enough.

Some argue that clinicians should treat AI as they do any complex tool—useful without needing to understand every detail of its operation. After all, few physicians can describe precisely how an MRI machine generates images, yet they interpret its output confidently. But this analogy is incomplete. An MRI produces a physical representation of anatomy based on well-understood principles of magnetism and resonance. It is a diagnostic aid, not a decision-maker. A black-box model, by contrast, *advises* or even *determines* clinical actions—without disclosing how it reached its judgment.

There is also a psychological dimension to consider. Trust in tools is not simply a matter of performance metrics. It is shaped by the ability to make sense of those tools. Studies have shown that clinicians are more likely to adopt AI systems when they can interrogate their outputs—ask *why*, not just *what*. Systems that are too confident, too opaque, or too inconsistent in their interface with human reasoning are often resisted—not because of arrogance or technophobia, but because responsible clinicians know what is at stake when decisions must be explained to a patient or defended to a review board.

Moreover, there is a pedagogical impact. If clinical reasoning is increasingly outsourced to models that do not explain themselves, what happens to the training of future doctors? Diagnostic acumen, like any cognitive skill, is honed through practice, reflection, and feedback. When models deliver answers without rationale, the opportunity for learning diminishes. The clinician becomes a passive recipient of outputs rather than an active participant in the interpretive process. The risk is not only the deskilling of individuals, but the erosion of a profession that has historically prized judgment as a mark of expertise.

Some developers are responding to these concerns by building "explainable AI" (XAI) systems—models designed to offer interpretable rationales alongside their predictions. These include heat maps for image analysis, feature importance rankings in structured data, and natural language explanations generated from decision trees. While promising, these approaches often involve trade-offs in performance, and there remains debate about whether post-hoc explanations are trustworthy or merely palatable simplifications. Transparency, it turns out, is not a technical fix. It is a sociotechnical challenge—requiring attention not only to algorithmic design, but to clinical culture, institutional norms, and the evolving demands of ethical care.

Perhaps the most important question is not whether AI can be made explainable, but whether medicine is willing to *slow down* enough to preserve the conditions in which explanation still matters. The drive toward automation, speed, and scale often assumes that faster decisions are better decisions. But good medicine is not merely efficient—it is *deliberate*. It recognises that some of the most important judgments are made not in the moment of diagnosis, but in the process of dialogue. A patient asks, "Why this treatment?" The doctor responds, "Because of these findings, this reasoning, and this experience." That exchange builds trust. It affirms agency. And it is precisely what is lost when the answer is, "Because the algorithm said so."

The future of clinical judgment in the age of black boxes will depend on more than model performance. It will depend on *designing systems that respect the epistemic commitments of medicine itself*: that decisions should be explainable, that trust should be earned through transparency, and that clinicians must remain accountable not only to outcomes, but to the people they serve. The challenge is not to choose between human reasoning and machine prediction, but to find a way to integrate them without erasing the very practices that make medicine humane. To do so, we must remember that care is not just what happens when we get the answer right. It is what happens when we are willing to explain why we chose it.

The Bias in the Machine

One of the great myths of artificial intelligence in medicine is that it functions above human prejudice—that by relying on data rather than personal judgment, it removes the distortions of bias, racism, sexism, and classism from healthcare. The reality is precisely the opposite. AI does not transcend bias; it *absorbs* it, processes it, and reproduces it—often at scale, often invisibly, and often under the guise of objectivity. The problem is not that the machine is malicious; it's that the machine is trained on a world that is.

At the heart of every AI model lies data: electronic health records, insurance claims, genomic sequences, patient surveys, and countless other sources. These data sets are not neutral archives. They are the residue of clinical decisions, institutional practices, and societal conditions—every one of which is shaped by historical inequalities. When a system learns from data, it is learning from a history of unequal access, unequal treatment, and unequal outcomes. It is learning from a world in which Black patients are less likely to receive pain medication, where women's cardiac symptoms are more likely to be misdiagnosed, where Indigenous patients are routinely undertreated, and where socioeconomic status predicts both illness and access to care with grim reliability.

Bias enters the machine at multiple points—not just in what data is used, but in *how* it is collected, *who* it represents, and *what* it is assumed to mean. If a predictive model is trained on hospital data from a population that is disproportionately white and affluent, then its conclusions will be most accurate for white, affluent patients. It may underperform, or misclassify entirely, when applied to people with different social, racial, or cultural backgrounds. This is not a technical glitch; it is a direct consequence of how health systems have historically documented—and distorted—the lives of marginalised groups.

The implications are not hypothetical. One widely publicised study published in *Science* in 2019 analysed an algorithm used by millions of patients in the United States to identify those in need of high-risk care management. The model was designed to allocate additional resources to patients predicted to be sicker in the future. But its proxy for sickness was healthcare spending. Because Black patients historically receive less care for the same conditions, they incurred lower costs—and were thus ranked as *less sick* than equally ill white patients. The model didn't encode race explicitly, but it encoded its effects. In doing so, it systematically deprived Black patients of access to enhanced care.

This is the insidious nature of algorithmic bias. It often functions through proxies—seemingly neutral variables that carry the imprint of structural inequality. Zip code stands in for income. Insurance status stands in for employment. Medication adherence stands in for social stability. These variables are not false; they are *contextually charged*. And when machine learning systems treat them as independent features rather than sociopolitical artefacts, they perpetuate a distorted image of who is at risk, who is compliant, who is deserving.

The problem deepens when these systems are deployed at scale and embedded into workflows. An algorithm used to triage emergency room patients may inadvertently de-prioritise non-English speakers, whose symptom descriptions do not match the patterns recognised by the model. A natural language processing tool trained on physician notes may learn to associate psychiatric diagnoses with terms more commonly used to describe women, thereby overpredicting mood disorders in female patients and underpredicting them in men. These are not hypothetical design flaws. They are real-world consequences of training machines on human systems that have always treated some patients as less credible, less complex, and less worth documenting in full.

Even the structure of data collection introduces bias. Electronic health records, while extensive, reflect what clinicians choose to document. And documentation is not a purely objective act—it is influenced by assumptions, time pressures, and unconscious stereotypes. A doctor may note "non-compliant" for a patient who missed appointments, but omit the fact that the patient lacked childcare or transport. A nurse may record "drug-seeking behaviour" without investigating chronic pain. Over time, these fragments accumulate into a dataset that appears factual, but is riddled with judgments masquerading as facts. And when that dataset becomes the foundation for predictive models, its biases become mathematically formalised.

It is tempting to imagine that technical adjustments—balancing training data, excluding protected attributes, applying fairness metrics—can solve the problem. These are important tools, but they are not cures. They treat the symptoms, not the cause. The deeper issue is epistemological: *what counts as knowledge in medicine*, and *whose experience is encoded in the data that machines are learning from*. In many cases, marginalised communities are not just underrepresented in training data—they are misrepresented, or not represented at all. The gaps are structural, not statistical.

The consequences for diagnostic and treatment outcomes are serious. A dermatology algorithm trained on images of light-skinned patients may fail to detect skin cancers in patients with darker skin tones. A cardiovascular risk calculator that does not account for the specific symptomatology of women may underestimate heart attack risk. A chatbot designed to support mental health may fail to recognise idioms of distress used by migrant populations or LGBTQ+ individuals, whose expressions of suffering deviate from dominant linguistic norms. These are not edge cases. They are evidence that *bias in training data is not an anomaly—it is the default condition of healthcare systems built in unequal societies.*

Addressing this requires more than technical refinement. It requires *political and institutional awareness.* It means acknowledging that AI systems are not deployed into a vacuum—they are inserted into clinical ecosystems shaped by long-standing disparities. If those systems are not critically examined, then AI will not mitigate bias. It will *accelerate it,* cloaked in the legitimacy of mathematical precision.

It also requires *rethinking what "good" data means.* In many current models, data quality is assessed by consistency, completeness, and scale. But a perfectly complete dataset that encodes racist clinical practices is not a solution—it is a liability. Instead, we must ask whether data captures *meaningful diversity,* whether it reflects the *lived realities* of those it aims to serve, and whether the *questions being asked* by the model are themselves equitable. For example, a model optimised to reduce cost per patient may improve efficiency while worsening outcomes for low-income patients who already receive less care. Optimisation is only as ethical as the objective function it serves.

Developing equitable AI in medicine will demand interdisciplinary collaboration. Clinicians, data scientists, social scientists, patients, and community advocates must be involved in model design—not as token stakeholders, but as co-creators. It will also demand transparency: who built the model, on what data, with what assumptions, and for whose benefit? Without this transparency, AI risks becoming a black box that not only hides its logic, but conceals the biases it reproduces.

Perhaps most urgently, it requires a moral imagination—a willingness to confront the uncomfortable truth that technology, no matter how advanced, cannot transcend the society that builds it. The promise of AI in healthcare will remain compromised until we reckon with the inequality in its foundations. That reckoning starts by refusing to treat bias as noise, and instead recognising it as signal—a signal of where our systems fail, who they overlook, and what must be reimagined if the future of medicine is to be just as well as precise.

Case Study: When AI Gets It Right—and Still Fails

A 54-year-old woman presents at a major metropolitan hospital with persistent fatigue, vague chest discomfort, and shortness of breath. She is soft-spoken, speaks English as a second language, and lives in a low-income, high-density housing complex. The emergency department, equipped with an AI-powered triage system, quickly processes her intake data: vital signs, past electronic health records, current complaints. The algorithm flags the case as "non-critical." Within minutes, the system sorts her into a lower-priority queue, optimising for throughput and clinical severity scores.

Twelve hours later, she returns in cardiac arrest. She had been having a heart attack all along—an atypical one. The AI did not "miss" the myocardial infarction in a clinical sense; it made a data-driven triage decision based on statistically common patterns. It performed exactly as trained. And yet, it failed. Not because it was inaccurate, but because it did not understand *her*.

This is not a parable. Variations of this case are documented in real healthcare systems deploying predictive triage tools. AI systems that excel in population-level accuracy can still collapse in the face of individual complexity. The failure, in these instances, is not technical—it is contextual. The model recognised disease patterns. It did not recognise personhood.

At the core of this problem is a tension that AI cannot resolve through greater computational power: *the disjunction between prediction and meaning*. Clinical algorithms are trained to detect statistical deviations from norms—to identify conditions, stratify risk, and recommend interventions. But what they fail to encode, and often cannot access, is the *narrative texture* of a patient's life. Language barriers, cultural expressions of pain, historical distrust of institutions, gendered assumptions about symptoms—these are not captured by biometric signals or diagnostic codes. Yet they shape the arc of illness and recovery with unrelenting force.

In another well-documented case from the United States, an AI-enabled diagnostic support system flagged a patient as high-risk for Type 2 diabetes based on biomarkers and behavioural indicators. The patient, a 45-year-old man from a Native American community, was indeed prediabetic. The system recommended an intensive lifestyle modification programme and flagged him for continuous monitoring. The data was "right." But the intervention failed entirely. The patient disengaged from care, became non-compliant by clinical standards, and eventually presented with severe complications.

When anthropologists were later consulted to understand the disconnect, they identified several factors the AI could not possibly have accounted for: the patient's cultural association of food with intergenerational trauma, a historical mistrust of institutional health programmes due to past abuses, and a local community framework in which individual health decisions are made collectively, not autonomously. The system had no interface for these forms of knowledge. It had no concept of what *caring well* would mean for that person, in that place, at that time.

What these cases illustrate is that *clinical correctness does not equal clinical adequacy*. A system can be functionally right and morally indifferent. This is particularly dangerous in healthcare, where the threshold for meaningful care is not mere detection of pathology, but the provision of care that aligns with a patient's values, context, and goals. A model trained on even the most sophisticated multi-modal data cannot infer whether a patient's distress is physical or existential. It cannot understand that declining an invasive treatment might be a rational choice rooted in religious belief, not medical ignorance.

This is not to suggest that AI cannot support or even enhance diagnostic precision. It can, and in many domains it already does. Algorithms now match or exceed human experts in radiology, dermatology, and oncology. But such success often relies on domains where inputs and outputs are bounded, where images can be labelled with clarity, and where disease presentation is relatively standardised. The further one moves into *complex, embodied, lived experience*, the less reliable these systems become—not in terms of processing power, but in terms of *clinical coherence*.

Failures of this kind are further complicated by the illusion of infallibility that often accompanies machine outputs. Clinicians, under pressure to deliver care at scale and speed, may over-trust algorithmic recommendations, especially when results are presented without uncertainty measures or interpretive rationale. In the first case, the junior physician who reviewed the triage flag trusted the system's non-urgent label, despite having a gut instinct that "something was off." With little time and an overburdened department, she deferred to the machine. That deference is not irrational—it is systemically conditioned. The problem is that it rests on a misplaced confidence: that what the model sees is all that matters.

And yet, the model sees *patterns*, not *people*. It sees risk scores, not relational history. It sees language features, not language nuance. When it "gets it right," it gets it right only within the frame it has been taught. And that frame, unless critically examined, remains startlingly narrow.

Some might argue that the solution is more data—more granular, more personal, more continuous. Wearables, ambient sensors, emotion-detection algorithms. But more data does not necessarily mean more understanding. In fact, it can create a *false sense of completeness*. In both cases above, the systems had access to vast data troves. What they lacked was interpretive context—*the kind of meaning that arises from conversation, trust, shared history, and cultural attunement.*

Others might argue that AI can be trained to detect such nuances—through better natural language processing, cross-cultural corpora, or multimodal data fusion. These are worthwhile efforts, but they come with epistemological limits. There is no dataset that captures grief in a dialect, or hesitation shaped by trauma. No label for "this symptom feels like something my mother had." No feature vector for dignity.

And so we return to a core proposition of this book: *AI may transform the infrastructure of care, but it cannot substitute for the moral and relational fabric that sustains healing.* A model that predicts disease but misses humanity has failed. Not computationally. *Clinically*.

It is tempting to celebrate the near-miraculous capabilities of medical AI—its speed, its scope, its power. But if we do so without asking what these systems *cannot* see, we risk a hollow form of progress. One in which patients are identified more accurately than ever before, and still misunderstood. One in which care becomes ever more precise, and still, somehow, less personal.

When AI gets it right and still fails, it exposes the thin line between detection and understanding. That line is the space of medicine. And unless it is safeguarded—not by better algorithms, but by better questions—we may find ourselves with a healthcare system that recognises the signal, but forgets the story.

Chapter 3
The Ethics of Prediction

A machine informs you that by the time you reach sixty-eight, you are likely to develop Alzheimer's. Not because of a symptom or a family history, but due to a pattern—some faint constellation of genomic markers, erratic sleep data, shifts in your speech cadence, the rhythm of your typing. You feel perfectly fine. And yet there it is: a 73.4 per cent probability, delivered with clinical precision. What do you do with such knowledge? What does your doctor do? Your insurer, your employer, your government, even the person you love—what will they do? Or rather, what should they be permitted to do?

This chapter begins at that uneasy crossroads where statistics collide with ethics. The moral landscape of prediction is no longer an academic curiosity; it is rapidly becoming one of the central dilemmas of modern medicine, public policy, and personal autonomy. Predictive algorithms have already slipped into the bloodstream of healthcare—risk calculators in emergency wards, AI triage systems, automated diagnostic aids in general practice. The revolution is not on the horizon; it has already arrived. The real question now is not *if* predictive medicine will transform healthcare, but *how* it will answer to the consequences of its own power.

Prediction, in its raw form, concerns probability. It is a language of likelihood, drawn from patterns and past outcomes. Responsibility, by contrast, belongs to the realm of *ought*—duty, conscience, moral weight. When a human clinician makes a decision, it is never merely mechanical; it carries ethical gravity because it arises from relationship—one person answerable to another, to their peers, to law, and to their own sense of right and wrong. When an AI system produces a risk score, that moral chain begins to fray. If harm results, who shoulders the blame? The doctor who trusted the model? The engineer who designed it? The hospital that purchased it? Or the patient who followed the advice? We are entering an age of what might be called distributed accountability—decision-making shared between human and machine, while responsibility evaporates into the gaps between them.

Consider, for instance, a London NHS Trust where a machine learning system flagged a patient as low-risk for sepsis. The clinician, reassured by the system's confidence, held off prescribing antibiotics. The patient deteriorated rapidly. Later reviews revealed that the model had underweighted several atypical biomarkers—outliers that, in this case, were decisive. When the family sought answers, the chain of accountability dissolved. The doctor blamed the algorithm. The developer blamed the data. The oversight committee blamed the absence of a clear policy. And in the end, no one bore the moral burden—except the family left behind.

Such stories are not mere exceptions. They signal a deeper, structural change. As predictive tools become enmeshed in clinical routines, the old moral architecture of medicine—anchored in discernment, judgement, and personal accountability—begins to warp. The "black box problem" is not just a technical riddle; it is an ethical one. When reasoning itself is concealed, moral agency slips into shadow.

Consent, once the crown jewel of medical ethics, is being quietly redefined. Informed consent presupposes that a patient can grasp what they are agreeing to: the purpose, risks, and alternatives of a proposed intervention. But what does it mean to consent to a *prediction*—an output derived not from causation but correlation, not from explanation but probability? And what of data consent, when the possible uses of that data are themselves unknowable at the moment of collection?

Imagine a woman using a fertility app. She consents to data tracking for one purpose: monitoring her ovulation. Years later, the app's parent company folds her anonymised information into a massive predictive model that estimates risk for postpartum depression. That model is then licensed to a private insurer, which quietly adjusts her premium. One day, she is denied a discount—not because she has a diagnosis, but because of what her data *suggests* she might one day become. She never agreed to that. Or did she, buried somewhere in a labyrinth of legal fine print?

This is the paradox of predictive consent. In a datafied world, consent is no longer a discrete moment—it is a continuous state of entanglement. Data flows, recombines, and learns without pause. Agency, in such a system, becomes porous. The individual is no longer simply consenting to a test or treatment, but to participation in a living network of algorithms whose implications may only emerge years later.

Privacy, too, has slipped its old definition. Once, it meant confidentiality—a closed file, a trusted doctor, a locked cabinet. Now, privacy concerns not only *who* accesses your data, but *what can be inferred* from it. A predictive model does not need your name to know you. It can infer your emotional state from your online tone, your stress levels from your typing speed, your potential depression from your late-night scrolling patterns. The surveillance here is not illicit—it is ambient, legal, and unseen.

Thus, predictive medicine creates a new kind of gaze: a surveillance that is anticipatory, not reactive. The promise is seductive—intervene early, prevent disease, save lives. Yet beneath that optimism lies a profound trade-off. If every life becomes a dataset, every body a potential risk factor, then healthcare risks becoming indistinguishable from monitoring. To be cared for is to be observed; to be observed is to be analysed; and analysis, inevitably, leads to judgment. The hospital morphs into a panopticon, the clinic into a quiet factory of prediction.

Nowhere is this more evident than in the rise of behavioural prediction. Algorithms now estimate not just who might get ill, but who might *comply*. They forecast which patients will take their medication, attend follow-ups, maintain diets. At first glance, this seems practical. But beneath the surface lies a moral conflation: between clinical risk and character. A missed appointment becomes a data point of unreliability; a poor diet becomes a signal of irresponsibility. Statistical profiling begins to shade into moral assessment.

These systems often claim neutrality, but prediction is never value-free. Every model encodes judgments—about normality, success, and failure. When a tool concludes that patients from a certain postcode are less likely to adhere to treatment, what follows? Are they offered more support, or quietly deprioritised? Does prediction serve equity, or does it codify inequality?

The ethics of prediction cannot be reduced to accuracy or efficiency. It concerns the very shape of medicine itself. A system that claims to know your future better than you do might indeed save lives—but it also risks constraining the human freedom to define one's own possibilities. Prediction, unexamined, becomes pre-emption; diagnosis, surveillance; care, control.

To grapple seriously with these tensions, we must move beyond the fascination with precision. We must ask: at what point does foresight become coercion? When does prevention begin to erode autonomy? Who, ultimately, benefits from predictive power—and who bears its cost?

This chapter traces those questions not as distant hypotheticals but as realities already unfolding. It seeks to rebuild the moral architecture of predictive healthcare—an architecture in which responsibility is not an afterthought but a foundation. For if prediction is to serve humanity, it must answer not only to data, but to dignity. Its challenge is not technical, but ethical. Its demand, not efficiency, but conscience.

Probability vs. Responsibility

A woman in her thirties enters an emergency room in Boston with nonspecific chest pain. An algorithm calculates her risk of cardiac arrest based on millions of data points culled from hospital records. The model returns a low probability—far below the intervention threshold. The attending physician, under pressure to discharge low-risk patients efficiently, follows the guidance. Six hours later, she returns in cardiac arrest. The algorithm, it turns out, was statistically correct: she was low risk *compared to the general population*. But to her, the outcome was binary—she either had a heart attack or she didn't. She did. The question that follows is not merely clinical. It is moral: *who is responsible?*

In predictive medicine, the boundary between statistical accuracy and ethical accountability is not just blurred—it is fundamentally misaligned. Probability deals in populations, in averages, in the tendencies of large groups. Responsibility, by contrast, is resolutely individual. It concerns the specific context of *this patient, this decision, this harm*. And as predictive systems proliferate in healthcare—delivering guidance on diagnoses, risk stratification, and treatment plans—the misalignment between these two domains becomes increasingly dangerous.

To understand this disjunction, we must first recognise that machine learning models are built to detect patterns that correlate with outcomes, not necessarily to explain them. When an algorithm trained on 100 million hospital visits identifies that patients over seventy with low blood pressure and high creatinine are at increased risk of renal failure, it does so without understanding physiology or pathophysiology. It observes patterns, not reasons. From a probability standpoint, it is often strikingly effective. From a responsibility standpoint, it is *indifferent*. A model does not weigh consequences. It does not consider harm. It does not ask, "Should this be done?" It asks, "What is likely to happen?"

This is where human moral frameworks begin to strain. Consider a scenario in which an algorithm predicts with high confidence that a patient with schizophrenia will not adhere to prescribed medication. A provider may then be prompted to reduce the complexity of care, or in some systems, limit treatment access based on predicted noncompliance. Statistically, this may be defensible. But ethically, it becomes deeply troubling. The patient is being pre-judged on the basis of group-level inference, not on their individual intent or circumstances. Probability is overriding personhood. *The risk becomes destiny.*

This dynamic produces a kind of *statistical fatalism*, where patients are treated not according to what they need, but according to what people like them *usually* do. In such a system, bias—especially when encoded in the training data—becomes a self-fulfilling prophecy. If historically, patients from certain ethnic or socioeconomic groups were less likely to receive certain interventions, a model trained on that data will "learn" that such patients are poor candidates for those treatments. And it will perpetuate the disparity in future recommendations—not out of malice, but out of mathematical fidelity to the past.

This reveals a central paradox of predictive healthcare: *An AI system can be both highly accurate and deeply unjust*. The model does what it was trained to do. The clinician, under time pressure and institutional incentives, may defer to the model. The system optimises for efficiency, not for equity. And yet when harm occurs, the moral vacuum becomes visible. Who is accountable? The algorithm? The developers? The data scientists who selected the training set? The institution that deployed the model? The doctor who clicked "approve"? Or the patient, whose life was shaped by a machine they could not interrogate?

Responsibility, in traditional medicine, is traceable. A physician makes a diagnosis, prescribes a treatment, follows a code of ethics, and is held accountable by licensure and litigation. There is a clear line of authority and liability. In algorithmically mediated care, this clarity erodes. The model is often a "black box"—its inner workings opaque even to its creators. Clinical decisions become a composite of human intuition and algorithmic suggestion, creating a grey zone where moral agency is diluted across systems. This is not an accident. It is an architectural feature of machine learning: *it distributes decision-making while diffusing responsibility*.

The problem is not just legal or procedural. It is *epistemological*. Algorithms alter how knowledge is produced in medicine. They recast the clinician not as an expert interpreter of signs and symptoms, but as an arbiter between competing probabilities. This changes the nature of care. In the probabilistic worldview, no decision is ever "right" or "wrong"—only more or less likely to succeed. But real patients live in the domain of consequences, not probabilities. They experience outcomes, not distributions.

There are attempts to address this with "explainable AI"—models that can offer human-readable justifications for their predictions. But even these systems often reduce to post hoc rationalisations rather than true causal insights. The ethical question remains: *Does explanation restore accountability, or merely perform it?* And if a clinician disagrees with a model, on what basis can they overrule it—especially when institutional protocols, insurance policies, or medico-legal pressures incentivise compliance with algorithmic guidance?

Take, for instance, the use of AI triage tools during the COVID-19 pandemic. Several hospitals implemented algorithms to allocate ventilators and ICU beds during periods of critical shortage. These models considered age, comorbidities, and likelihood of recovery. But embedded within these calculations were assumptions about quality of life, productivity, and social value—assumptions that often mirrored societal biases. Elderly patients, disabled individuals, and those with chronic mental illness were sometimes deprioritised. The models were efficient. But were they just?

These tensions demand more than technical safeguards. They require a philosophical reckoning. *What is the ethical status of a probability?* Does a 92% likelihood absolve a decision-maker from responsibility when harm occurs in the 8%? If we allow models to inform decisions that carry life-altering consequences, we must also define the moral and legal frameworks under which those decisions are made.

A truly responsible system would require transparency not just in how models work, but in *who is accountable when they don't.* It would offer patients recourse not merely when rules are broken, but when predictions cause harm—even if the system worked "as intended." It would empower clinicians to exercise judgement *in dialogue* with prediction, rather than as its subordinate. And it would resist the seduction of algorithmic certainty, recognising that *the appearance of objectivity is not the same as the presence of justice.*

Responsibility in predictive healthcare must be redefined as a collective enterprise—but not a diffuse one. Clarity is essential. Developers must own the assumptions they bake into models. Institutions must audit the outcomes these models produce. Regulators must set standards not just for accuracy, but for fairness and harm mitigation. And clinicians must retain the moral courage to interrogate outputs, not merely implement them.

Most importantly, patients must be treated as agents, not datapoints. Their experiences, values, and narratives must matter—not just because they humanise care, but because they *resist the flattening force of probability*. Every prediction must be tempered by the question: *what does this mean for this person, in this moment, with this history?*

Until that question is central, predictive systems will continue to function with statistical brilliance and moral opacity. And the cost of that disjunction will be borne by those whose lives are reduced to likelihoods.

Consent in a Predictive World

When a patient signs a consent form before surgery or agrees to have their blood drawn for testing, the ethical architecture underpinning that act is relatively stable: there is a procedure, a risk, an individual decision. The stakes are immediate, the consequences foreseeable. But what does consent mean when a person's heartbeat is continuously monitored by a wearable device, when their search history feeds into a model predicting the onset of depression, or when decades of digitised health records quietly inform a future clinical recommendation? *In predictive healthcare, the very nature of consent is under strain—not because patients are unwilling, but because they are increasingly unable to understand what they are consenting to.*

The challenge is not simply one of legal formality or procedural ethics. It is epistemic. The core principle of informed consent—first articulated in the aftermath of World War II and later codified in bioethics—is that patients must be given sufficient understanding to make autonomous decisions about their own care. But in the predictive paradigm, where data is repurposed, recombined, and analysed in ways that are neither visible nor comprehensible to the average person, *true understanding becomes elusive.* The gap between what patients think they are authorising and what is actually happening to their data has widened into a chasm.

Consider the case of predictive modelling for hospital readmission. A seemingly innocuous dataset—a patient's vital signs, medication history, and lab results—is fed into a proprietary algorithm to forecast the probability of that patient returning within 30 days. The model's output may influence discharge planning, access to post-acute care services, or even insurance reimbursement. But nowhere in this process is the patient likely to be explicitly told: *Your risk score might affect whether we prioritise your follow-up care.* More importantly, even if told, could they fully grasp the implications? *Consent, in this context, becomes procedural theatre—formally obtained, substantively hollow.*

There is a particular irony here. The more sophisticated our data systems become, the more opaque their consequences. Predictive analytics does not merely track; it shapes. It turns future possibilities into present-day decisions. It assigns risk, not neutrally, but consequentially. If a patient is flagged as high risk for opioid misuse based on behavioural correlates, a physician may be discouraged from prescribing pain relief—even if the individual patient has never exhibited any signs of misuse. The data prediction, however probabilistic, begins to exert *prescriptive* force. And yet the patient has likely never been asked: *Do you consent to having your risk profile—generated by historical data of people you have never met—determine how we treat your pain?*

This is not a matter of conspiratorial intent or institutional malice. It is the product of a healthcare system that has become entangled with digital infrastructure designed around scale, efficiency, and optimisation. *Consent, in such systems, is often designed for compliance, not comprehension.* Terms and conditions run to thousands of words. Language is abstract and technical. Consent is obtained once, but data is reused indefinitely. The logic of the platform economy—familiar from social media and e-commerce—has migrated into clinical environments, but without the same regulatory scrutiny or public debate.

Even when patients are told that their data may be used for research, quality improvement, or predictive analytics, they are rarely in a position to appreciate the scope or the stakes. In practice, "broad consent" models authorise the use of health data for a potentially unlimited array of secondary purposes. A blood sample given for cholesterol testing today may contribute to an algorithm that predicts mental health deterioration years later. Data extracted from an electronic health record may end up training models that are sold to private companies or deployed in contexts entirely unrelated to the original clinical interaction. *The patient's body becomes a data asset—but the patient remains epistemically excluded from the processes their data fuels.*

There is a growing movement within bioethics and data governance circles to reimagine consent not as a single moment of authorisation but as an ongoing relationship—one that is transparent, dialogical, and responsive. Dynamic consent platforms, for example, allow patients to set granular preferences and receive updates on how their data is used. In theory, these systems could restore some measure of agency. But in practice, they remain underdeveloped, underfunded, and largely peripheral to mainstream healthcare infrastructure. Moreover, they require high levels of digital literacy and sustained engagement—luxuries not available to all patients equally.

This brings us to a deeper point: *consent is not merely a procedural checkbox; it is a function of power.* When systems are designed in ways that privilege institutional interests, technological complexity, and commercial opacity, the capacity of individuals to exercise informed choice is systematically undermined. The fiction of consent is maintained, but its ethical substance is hollowed out.

There are particular concerns when predictive analytics intersect with populations that are already structurally disadvantaged. Migrant patients, for example, may have limited understanding of local health systems or data governance frameworks. Patients from lower socioeconomic backgrounds may face language barriers or be subject to implicit coercion—believing that refusal to share data might compromise their care. In these contexts, *"consent" may be little more than acquiescence under constrained conditions.*

The problem is compounded when predictive systems move from forecasting disease to inferring behaviour. Models that estimate the likelihood of medication adherence, lifestyle change, or mental health relapse do not merely reflect biology; they render judgement. They convert personal history, social context, and behavioural variance into risk metrics. The individual is reframed as a statistical profile—and often without being asked. A patient may be scored as "noncompliant" based on prior missed appointments, financial instability, or even the tone of clinician notes in an EHR. These data points are not inherently predictive; they are interpreted as such by systems that lack contextual understanding. Yet decisions may be made on this basis, with the patient never informed, never consulted, never invited to challenge the classification.

This shift from *consent to be treated* to *consent to be predicted* marks a profound transformation in the ethics of medicine. It raises urgent questions: Is consent meaningful when patients don't know what models are making inferences about them? Should there be a right not to be predicted? Should patients be notified when predictions about their health, behaviour, or mortality are being made—especially when these predictions carry actionable consequences? And perhaps most importantly, who bears responsibility when predictions based on consented data result in harm?

Legal scholars have begun to grapple with these dilemmas, pointing out that current data protection laws, such as GDPR in the European context, provide limited safeguards in clinical environments where predictive modelling is treated as a "healthcare function." There is growing recognition that *privacy rights and consent mechanisms must be retooled for a world in which data does not merely document the present but constructs the future.* Yet the regulatory frameworks remain reactive, fragmented, and often lag behind technological deployment.

Ultimately, the challenge of consent in a predictive world is not just to ensure that patients *agree*—it is to ensure that they *understand what they are agreeing to.* This will require more than improved language or simplified forms. It will require a rethinking of the moral relationship between patients and the systems that interpret them. Consent must move from a formality to a practice; from a contract to a conversation; from an institutional safeguard to a genuine expression of autonomy.

Until then, the ethical legitimacy of predictive healthcare remains compromised—not because its predictions are inaccurate, but because they operate in the absence of truly informed permission. A system that knows more about patients than patients know about the system cannot claim to be morally transparent. It can only claim to be efficient. And that is not enough.

Privacy in the Age of Proactive Surveillance

A smartwatch doesn't feel like a surveillance device. Nor does a fitness app, a menstrual tracker, or an always-on blood glucose monitor. These tools speak the language of empowerment—"Know your body," "Own your health," "Prevent disease before it starts." Yet beneath the sleek interfaces and wellness slogans lies a far less visible architecture: *a system of continuous data extraction that reframes healthcare as a project of proactive surveillance.* It is a shift that promises earlier intervention, personalised insight, and optimised outcomes. But it also reconfigures the boundaries of privacy, agency, and clinical responsibility in ways that remain underexamined—and increasingly consequential.

Unlike traditional healthcare encounters, which are episodic and bounded by clinical context, the logic of continuous monitoring is ambient, ambient and often ambiently coercive. It operates in the background, turning physiological processes into constant streams of analysable data—sleep cycles, heart rhythms, cortisol levels, blood oxygen, steps taken, calories burned, hours of screen time, even vocal tone and keyboard cadence. What was once private, biological, and internal becomes externalised, objectified, and machine-readable. *The body is no longer simply cared for—it is watched.*

This shift is not purely technological. It is cultural and conceptual. It marks a transition from *reactive care,* in which the clinical system responds to symptoms, to *proactive management,* in which risk itself becomes the object of intervention. In this paradigm, *data precedes illness.* Predictive analytics aims not only to treat but to anticipate, to detect precursors to disease before they emerge, to intervene before the patient knows there's anything wrong. Surveillance is no longer an exception triggered by clinical suspicion; it is the new default.

The implications for privacy are profound, not because monitoring is covert, but because it is normalised. When surveillance is voluntary, incentivised, or presented as care, it bypasses traditional defences. A person who would never agree to share their heart rate with an insurance company may do so through a fitness app tied to a reward scheme. A parent concerned about their child's digital footprint may consent to school-based behavioural tracking software, reassured by promises of mental health support. *The surveillance becomes embedded within care, cloaked in benevolence, and thus escapes scrutiny.*

And yet, this care-surveillance fusion introduces new vulnerabilities. Consider the case of a workplace wellness programme that encourages employees to wear biometric devices in exchange for lower insurance premiums. Ostensibly voluntary, such programmes carry implicit pressure: those who opt out may be perceived as uncooperative, while those who participate relinquish ongoing access to behavioural data—sleep, exercise, stress. Over time, this data may inform performance evaluations, absence reviews, or even hiring decisions. What began as self-care morphs into managerial oversight.

In clinical settings, similar dynamics unfold. Hospitals increasingly deploy remote monitoring systems for post-operative patients, chronic disease management, or mental health tracking. These systems offer clear benefits: early detection of complications, reduced readmissions, improved adherence. But they also raise critical questions. What happens when a patient's data signals noncompliance—erratic medication use, poor sleep, missed physiotherapy sessions? Who decides whether these deviations are medical concerns, lifestyle choices, or grounds for intervention? *And how much insight does the patient have into how these signals are interpreted, shared, and acted upon?*

The broader risk is not just that individuals are being monitored—it is that they are being *interpreted* by systems whose logic they cannot see, let alone contest. The data captured by wearables and health apps is often fed into proprietary algorithms—"black boxes" that generate risk scores, behavioural flags, or clinical alerts without explaining their rationale. This opacity undermines informed consent and accountability. A person flagged as at-risk for cardiac events may not know why. A mental health patient may be subjected to intensified monitoring based on correlations they never authorised. *When the interpretation of data is outsourced to opaque models, privacy is eroded not only in content but in control.*

Moreover, the line between medical and non-medical surveillance is increasingly blurred. Many of the companies developing health monitoring tools are not healthcare providers but technology firms whose primary revenue model is data monetisation. The legal protections for health data—such as HIPAA in the United States or GDPR in Europe—apply narrowly and inconsistently. A heart rate collected in a hospital is governed by one set of rules; the same data collected by a consumer device may be subject to entirely different standards, or none at all. *Functionally identical data flows through radically unequal regimes of accountability.*

The result is a fragmented landscape in which patients and users are left to navigate their privacy on their own—often with little guidance, limited recourse, and a deep asymmetry of knowledge. Even when privacy policies are disclosed, they are rarely read or understood. The language is dense, the implications unclear, and the options limited. Opting out often means foregoing services, benefits, or insights. Privacy becomes a privilege rather than a right—available only to those with the time, literacy, and leverage to resist.

And this surveillance does not affect everyone equally. People from marginalised communities—racial minorities, disabled individuals, those with mental illness or substance use histories—are more likely to be subjected to intensive monitoring. Predictive models trained on biased datasets may overstate their risk, flag their behaviour as aberrant, or assign them to high-surveillance categories. Once flagged, they are more likely to face restrictive interventions, suspicion, or denial of care. *Surveillance, in practice, amplifies social inequity—under the banner of proactive health.*

There are also psychological dimensions to this transformation. Living under constant biometric observation can induce self-regulation, anxiety, or compulsive tracking. People may feel obligated to meet arbitrary goals—10,000 steps, 8 hours of sleep, a perfectly stable heart rate—not because they are clinically necessary, but because the device expects it. This gamification of health can displace intuition and autonomy. Individuals may start to believe their wellness is only real when validated by data. *The body is experienced less as lived, and more as measured.*

Defenders of proactive surveillance rightly point to its life-saving potential. Wearables can detect atrial fibrillation, alert users to abnormal glucose trends, or provide early signs of relapse in patients with bipolar disorder. But the benefits are uneven, and the trade-offs underexplored. The capacity to monitor does not inherently confer the wisdom to intervene. Nor does it justify the erosion of fundamental rights. *A just healthcare system must distinguish between care that informs and surveillance that controls.*

If proactive monitoring is to become a cornerstone of future medicine—and that outcome seems likely—then its governance must be reimagined. First, there must be transparency: patients should know what is being monitored, by whom, and for what purpose. Second, consent must be specific, revocable, and contextual. Third, data access must be equitable and non-punitive. Refusal to participate in monitoring should not entail diminished care. Fourth, interpretability must be prioritised. People have a right to understand how data about them is used to draw conclusions about them. *Opacity may be efficient for systems, but it is corrosive to trust.*

Finally, there must be robust oversight—not only from regulatory bodies but from ethics boards, patient advocacy groups, and affected communities. The decisions about when, how, and why to monitor should not be left to technologists or market incentives alone. *Healthcare is not a surveillance industry with a humanistic front; it is a moral enterprise grounded in dignity, autonomy, and justice.*

The age of proactive surveillance is not an aberration—it is the shape of healthcare to come. Its trajectory is neither wholly dystopian nor entirely redemptive. But its stakes are high, and its impact already unfolding. The challenge is not to resist technology, but to *demand governance that respects the boundary between care and control*. Privacy is not a sentimental ideal or a bureaucratic hurdle. It is the precondition for meaningful trust in a system that increasingly knows us better than we know ourselves. And that trust, once lost, cannot be recovered through convenience or speed. It must be earned—through transparency, fairness, and an unwavering commitment to human dignity in the face of machine efficiency.

Predicting Behavior, Not Just Biology

A patient's blood pressure can be measured in millimetres of mercury. Their weight, heart rate, cholesterol, and glucose can be tracked with near-clinical precision. But will they remember to take their medication? Will they exercise three times a week as advised? Will they attend follow-up appointments or change their diet in response to risk scores? These are not biochemical questions—they are behavioural ones. And increasingly, they are being modelled, predicted, and acted upon by algorithmic systems that *presume to know not just what the body will do, but what the person will choose.*

Healthcare has long sought ways to account for the unpredictability of human behaviour. Patients skip pills, ignore advice, lie about drinking, and resist lifestyle change even when confronted with compelling evidence. These deviations from clinical rationality are not mere outliers—they are part of the reality of care. Traditionally, clinicians addressed them through relationships: understanding why a patient hesitates, working with their values, constraints, and ambivalence. But as data-driven tools gain ground, a new paradigm is emerging—*behavioural prediction as a proxy for responsibility*. The model doesn't need to ask why; it only needs to forecast what will happen next.

This shift is subtle but consequential. Predictive models now estimate a patient's likelihood of adhering to a medication regimen, following discharge instructions, showing up for mental health appointments, or responding to behavioural nudges. These predictions are derived not from clinical insight, but from patterns in demographic, behavioural, and sometimes non-medical data—postal codes, previous appointment histories, shopping habits, online behaviour, or even credit scores. *What was once understood as personal context becomes a statistical signal.* And once that signal exists, systems begin to act on it.

Consider a hospital system using a model to predict which discharged patients are least likely to adhere to follow-up care. Those flagged as "high risk" may receive extra reminders or support services—a seemingly benign and even beneficial intervention. But they may also be deprioritised for certain treatments, referred to social services instead of specialists, or face more paternalistic clinical encounters. *Risk becomes a label that follows the patient, not simply a guide to care.*

What makes this evolution particularly complex is that behavioural prediction doesn't merely describe—it *judges*. A patient predicted to miss appointments may be labelled noncompliant. One flagged for low adherence may be seen as careless. These judgments are rarely explicit, but they shape how clinicians allocate attention, time, and trust. And unlike biological predictions—which are understood to be probabilistic—behavioural predictions tend to carry moral weight. *We are more forgiving of a failing heart than a failing will.*

This moralisation of behaviour through data introduces a subtle but profound shift in the ethics of care. In traditional clinical practice, judgment was situated within relationships. A clinician might know a patient struggles to adhere because they are caring for an ill spouse, working two jobs, or managing anxiety. That insight would shape the plan. But when prediction replaces interpretation, *the why is stripped away, and only the risk remains.* The model does not care whether a person misses pills because of financial stress or forgetfulness. It only cares that they miss them—and it calibrates future expectations accordingly.

These models are not neutral. Their outputs are shaped by their inputs, and those inputs are shaped by systemic inequalities. A Black woman with limited access to pharmacies, variable employment, and a history of distrust in the healthcare system may be flagged as high-risk for nonadherence—not because of personal failing, but because the system has repeatedly failed her. Yet the model does not distinguish structural disadvantage from individual disposition. *It flattens biography into behaviour, and behaviour into liability.*

The implications extend beyond individual care. Behavioural prediction is being used to inform population-level strategies, such as risk-based insurance pricing, triage prioritisation, and preventive outreach. Health insurers use lifestyle scores to determine premiums. Pharmaceutical companies target "high-adherence" patients for drug trials. Employers assess wellness programme eligibility based on predicted engagement. *In each case, the model does not just predict what people will do—it shapes what they are offered, how they are seen, and how their care is configured.*

These developments challenge the ethical foundations of consent and autonomy. Can a patient meaningfully consent to treatment if they are unaware that a behavioural score is shaping the options presented to them? Can clinicians trust that risk predictions reflect genuine need, or are they reflecting biases embedded in the data? Who is accountable when a patient's care is altered—or denied—based on an algorithmic assumption about their future actions?

There is also the matter of feedback loops. If a patient is predicted to be noncompliant and therefore given less complex treatment, lower dosages, or less clinician engagement, the model's forecast may become self-fulfilling. The person's health outcomes decline—not because of their behaviour, but because of the care they were not offered. Over time, these dynamics reinforce disparities, entrench stigma, and harden the very inequalities that predictive systems claim to mitigate. *Prediction becomes prophecy.*

Defenders of behavioural modelling argue that such systems enable targeted intervention, efficient resource use, and improved outcomes. And there is truth to this. Not all patients need the same kind of care. Understanding who is most at risk of disengagement can inform better support, smarter outreach, and more personalised engagement strategies. But this promise depends entirely on *how* the predictions are used—and whether their use is transparent, fair, and respectful of patients as moral agents, not just behavioural probabilities.

The challenge, then, is not whether behavioural prediction should exist—it already does. The question is how to ensure it serves care, rather than control. This requires rethinking both the design and deployment of predictive tools. First, systems must prioritise interpretability: patients and clinicians should understand what a score means, how it was generated, and how it will be used. Second, there must be accountability: when predictions shape access to care, there must be mechanisms to question, contest, or override them. Third, equity must be baked into the modelling process: datasets must be audited for bias, and outcomes monitored for disparate impact.

But perhaps most importantly, *the logic of behavioural prediction must be kept in its place.* It is a tool, not a truth. A probability, not a person. It cannot replace the clinical conversation, the ethical negotiation, the listening and responding that makes care more than calculation. A model can predict that someone won't take their pills. Only a person can ask *why*, and offer help.

As predictive systems grow more powerful, the temptation will be to treat behaviour as just another variable to optimise—alongside blood pressure and BMI. But behaviour is different. It is shaped by history, culture, psychology, and circumstance. To predict it without understanding it is not care; it is *control masquerading as efficiency.* And to act on those predictions without reflection is to risk replacing clinical wisdom with algorithmic overreach.

In the end, the move to model behaviour marks a crossing point in healthcare's transformation. It signals not just a new frontier of data, but a new kind of judgment—one that no longer comes from a conversation between two people, but from a silent calculation behind the scenes. Whether that judgment serves the patient or the system depends on the choices we make now—about transparency, ethics, governance, and the enduring value of treating people not just as bodies to be cured or behaviours to be managed, but as persons to be understood.

Chapter 4
When the System Speaks for You

A patient arrives at the emergency department—breath short, thoughts scattered, words faltering. Before a single question leaves the clinician's mouth, an algorithm has already spoken. It has assigned a triage score, ranked their urgency, and concluded that their condition is non-critical. In a system engineered for efficiency, that score becomes their surrogate—standing in for their story, their distress, their right to be heard. The machine has spoken, and in the quiet authority of its output, the patient's own voice fades into the background.

That a system might "speak" for a person is no longer a metaphor. In contemporary healthcare, AI systems routinely mediate access to care, shape priorities, and recommend treatments—all before a human interaction even begins. From emergency triage to chronic care management, from mental health assessments to telehealth routing, decisions that once relied on conversation and judgement are increasingly automated. These systems do not merely assist clinicians; they begin to *replace* the interpretive act itself.

Advocates insist this is progress—less bias, greater speed, fewer errors. And, within limits, they are right. On tightly defined tasks, machine precision can indeed outstrip human judgement. But there is a threshold at which automation crosses from assistance into substitution, when the system begins to *speak for* the patient rather than *with* them. The difference is profound. A statistical model, no matter how advanced, does not ask what the patient values. It cannot detect irony, trauma, or hesitation. It does not know how to question its own certainty. It declares. And its declarations often carry the weight of finality.

This chapter examines what is at stake—what is muted, and who becomes inaudible—when algorithmic systems claim the right to speak. It explores how automation quietly transforms advocacy into proxy, and how computational certainty begins to displace the uncertainty that once made medicine humane. It also places predictive modelling alongside narrative medicine, contrasting the world of probabilities with the world of stories. At heart, this is not just a technical dispute—it is a question of knowledge. What counts as truth when lived experience is translated into data?

At the centre lies a contradiction: the tools that promise personalisation often enact erasure. A model trained on aggregated data can only recognise what recurs; it cannot register what resists pattern. In doing so, it amplifies majority narratives while dimming those on the margins. It listens not to the person, but to history—and history, as medicine well knows, is far from neutral.

Take, for instance, the chronic underestimation of pain among Black patients. For decades, clinical records have reflected this disparity. Now, when AI systems are trained on those same records, they perpetuate the error, but at scale. Bias is reborn as data. Objectivity becomes its disguise. A patient's suffering is filtered through inherited silence, transmuted into a number that claims to know.

The danger intensifies for those whose illnesses defy neat classification—patients with autoimmune disorders, chronic fatigue, or complex trauma. Their conditions resist quantification; their healing depends on narrative space. Predictive systems, however, parse only what they can measure. A long pause becomes a marker of mental instability. Missed appointments become evidence of noncompliance. An outlier reading becomes noise. Thus, the patient's voice is not only neglected—it is overwritten by code.

Even the language of these systems carries an aura of inevitability. Risk scores. Confidence intervals. Decision trees. Presented on a screen, they look impartial, mathematical, incontrovertible. But each one reflects choices—design assumptions, institutional pressures, data boundaries. When clinicians, pressed for time, are presented with such outputs, they may internalise their authority. The machine's voice grows louder, and the clinician's intuition fainter. Eventually, both are drowned out by the hum of the system.

The consequences reach far beyond individual errors. As automated triage and recommendation tools proliferate, the moral architecture of medicine begins to shift. When a patient is deprioritised because an algorithm misreads atypical symptoms—say, a woman experiencing a heart attack without chest pain—who answers for the oversight? The clinician who followed the recommendation? The data scientists? The institution? Responsibility, once anchored in human judgement, now diffuses across code, protocol, and machine output.

These are not hypothetical anxieties. In documented cases across several health systems, patients have been harmed—sometimes fatally—because predictive tools failed to recognise nuance. The explanations are often elusive. "The model made the call," one might hear. But no one can say precisely why. The story, in the end, remains unread.

Yet beneath the technical failures lies a deeper philosophical fracture: the difference between being spoken for and being heard. The first implies substitution; the second, recognition. The finest traditions of medicine have always privileged listening as a moral act. Narrative medicine, in particular, teaches that meaning emerges through dialogue—through fragments, gestures, silences. It allows for uncertainty, even contradiction. It reminds us that a patient is not a problem to be solved, but a person to be understood.

In contrast, predictive systems leave no room for such ambiguity. They do not wait to listen; they calculate. The patient ceases to be narrator and becomes instead a source of input—a case, a dataset, a row in a spreadsheet. The clinician, pressured by time and reassured by automation, follows suit. The machine's confidence becomes contagious.

This is not an argument for rejecting AI in medicine. The question is not whether machines should assist us, but how far they should speak in our place. A system that claims to understand without truly *knowing*—that performs empathy without experiencing it—commits a subtle betrayal. And when institutions equate automation with progress, they risk constructing an architecture of silence, where care becomes indistinguishable from compliance.

The challenge, then, is threefold: ethical, political, epistemic. We must ask what voices our data privileges, what biases our systems perpetuate, and how to preserve the act of listening as a clinical and moral practice. How can we design technologies that amplify the patient's story instead of compressing it into metrics? How do we ensure that systems built to assist do not become the arbiters of truth?

This chapter turns to those questions. Through lived cases and conceptual reflection, it traces how the algorithm's voice has risen to prominence—and what must be done to restore the primacy of the patient's own.

The Automation of Advocacy

When a patient seeks medical attention, their most urgent need is not simply treatment but *representation*. They need to be seen, heard, and interpreted—not as a composite of symptoms, but as a human being whose life context shapes the meaning of their condition. Historically, this interpretive task has belonged to clinicians: general practitioners, emergency doctors, nurses, and social workers whose judgments emerged from conversation, observation, and experience. Today, however, an increasing share of that representational work has been outsourced—not to other humans, but to machines. As artificial intelligence systems assume roles in triage, resource allocation, and care pathway decisions, they are no longer just analytical tools; they are becoming *proxies*—technological stand-ins for patients in moments where advocacy can mean the difference between care and neglect, relief and harm, dignity and dismissal.

The rise of AI as patient proxy is not a hypothetical trend. In numerous health systems across the globe, predictive triage algorithms now rank patients in real time based on expected acuity. Emergency departments in the UK and US routinely deploy risk-scoring tools to assess who should be seen first, who can wait, and who should be redirected. Health insurers in the private sector are using behavioural prediction models to determine the probability of future hospitalisation, shaping access to interventions before a patient has even presented symptoms. Triage bots, decision support software, and automated referral engines now influence clinical workflows at multiple junctures. And in doing so, they are increasingly tasked with the function of advocacy—*speaking on behalf of the patient to determine what happens next.*

This shift is both technically sophisticated and ethically volatile. At its core is a fundamental reframing of advocacy from an interpretive, context-sensitive relationship into a computational optimisation problem. Traditional clinical advocacy is grounded in an ethic of listening: understanding not just what is wrong with a person, but what matters to them. It is responsive, situated, and accountable. By contrast, algorithmic advocacy is governed by predictive logic—it relies on patterns derived from historical data, expressed through probability scores, risk categories, and decision trees. *It does not hear; it estimates.*

And herein lies the core tension: while predictive systems may be more consistent or efficient in some scenarios, they are inherently incapable of responding to human nuance in the way that meaningful advocacy demands. For example, a triage model may determine that a patient with stable vital signs and a recorded history of anxiety does not require urgent attention. Yet it may miss the fact that their current episode is qualitatively different, tied to a recent trauma, or that their reluctance to fully disclose symptoms stems from past experiences of dismissal. A human clinician, attuned to subtle cues—hesitation, body language, emotional tone—might investigate further. The algorithm, having been trained on input-output pairs and optimisation thresholds, does not pause for reconsideration. It speaks through classification, not curiosity.

This is not to suggest that human judgment is infallible. Indeed, many of the systems now in use were developed precisely because of concerns about inconsistency, implicit bias, or overburdened decision-making. But replacing flawed judgment with opaque automation merely displaces the problem. In many cases, AI systems *inherit* the biases embedded in the data they were trained on, while simultaneously reducing transparency and eliminating recourse. When a machine misrepresents a patient, there is often no appeal—no space for dialogue, explanation, or dissent. *The patient becomes the product of a decision process they cannot interrogate.*

Consider the case of a Medicaid management company in the United States that used an AI tool to identify "high-cost" patients for proactive outreach and care coordination. The model correctly identified individuals with frequent hospital visits and complex comorbidities. But when auditors investigated, they found a troubling pattern: Black patients with the same level of clinical risk were consistently ranked lower than their white counterparts. Why? Because the algorithm used *cost* as a proxy for *need*—and Black patients, due to structural inequities, historically received less care, even when they were sicker. Thus, the system's advocacy was skewed: it amplified existing disparities rather than correcting them. *It spoke, but not truthfully.*

Another example emerged in the use of AI-driven symptom checkers, deployed during the COVID-19 pandemic. In several countries, these tools were promoted as first-line triage aids to reduce hospital load. Yet multiple evaluations found that these bots under-prioritised women and ethnic minorities, particularly when symptoms were non-standard or described in culturally inflected language. A woman experiencing fatigue, body aches, and shortness of breath—symptoms not uncommon in cardiac events—might be told to self-monitor at home, while a man describing chest tightness might be directed to emergency care. In this scenario, the system's voice shapes not just perception, but action. It stands in for a clinician's judgment, often without sufficient evidence or accountability. *Its silence is not neutral.*

The automation of advocacy also brings with it a transformation of power dynamics in clinical environments. As algorithms increasingly mediate between patients and clinicians, they recalibrate who gets to speak and who is listened to. A clinician presented with a machine-generated "recommendation" may feel pressure—implicit or explicit—to defer to it, especially when institutional policies reward compliance with AI guidance. This deference is not always a matter of trust; it is often about liability, efficiency, and systemic inertia. *The system is designed to be followed, not questioned.*

Yet even as these systems proliferate, the conceptual framework to govern them remains underdeveloped. What does it mean for a machine to "advocate"? Can an algorithm meaningfully act in the best interest of a person it cannot understand? If advocacy requires empathy, moral reasoning, and contextual sensitivity—qualities beyond the scope of current machine intelligence—then what are we really automating? *Not advocacy, but decision-making disguised as care.*

The implications are profound. At stake is not simply the technical accuracy of AI tools, but the moral architecture of medicine. If we delegate the act of speaking for patients to systems that cannot feel, reflect, or be held to account, we risk hollowing out the core ethic of care. We also risk normalising a healthcare landscape in which people are represented by proxies they did not choose, in processes they do not understand, with outcomes they cannot challenge. This is not a dystopian projection; it is a creeping reality already embedded in triage algorithms, remote monitoring platforms, and clinical workflow optimisers. *Advocacy becomes automation, and automation becomes authority.*

To respond responsibly, we must resist the framing of these systems as neutral or inevitable. We must ask: Who designs the proxy? Whose voices are encoded in its training data? What values govern its decisions? And most importantly, how do we preserve the space for human representation when systems are built to replace it? Answering these questions requires not just technical audits, but *ethical scrutiny, interdisciplinary dialogue, and structural reform.*

There is, perhaps, a place for systems that assist in advocacy—tools that highlight overlooked symptoms, surface patient-reported concerns, or flag discrepancies between observed data and stated experience. But these tools must be subordinate to human relationships, not superior to them. They must be accountable, interrogable, and context-aware. They must augment voice, not displace it.

Ultimately, the automation of advocacy poses a challenge that transcends healthcare: it asks us what it means to speak for someone with integrity. Whether in triage decisions or policy algorithms, the question is the same: When we build systems to act on behalf of others, how do we ensure they remain servants of human dignity, rather than substitutes for it? The answer will not be found in code alone. It will be found in how we choose to listen, even when it is faster not to.

Voice, Silence, and Marginalisation

In healthcare, silence is rarely neutral. It is not simply the absence of speech, but often the product of power—of whose pain is recognised, whose symptoms are believed, whose experiences are encoded into diagnostic frameworks. When medical artificial intelligence is trained on historical data, it does not just learn medicine; it learns *medicine as it has been practised*—complete with all its embedded inequities, omissions, and patterns of disregard. The result is that algorithmic systems, hailed as objective and impartial, can quietly amplify the very exclusions they were meant to overcome. *They do not just reflect bias—they perpetuate silence where voice was already missing.*

To understand how this occurs, consider the foundational logic of machine learning: pattern recognition derived from past data. If certain populations—women, ethnic minorities, neurodivergent patients, transgender individuals—have historically been underdiagnosed, misdiagnosed, or dismissed in clinical settings, then their health experiences are underrepresented in the datasets that feed these systems. That absence is not benign. It means that AI tools may fail to detect conditions that manifest differently across populations, overlook symptoms described in culturally distinct ways, or ignore emerging health issues that are not yet statistically "proven." *The algorithm listens to the data it has been given, and ignores what has never been said.*

This silence has consequences not just for diagnosis, but for belief. Take, for instance, the long history of women reporting pain that is minimised or psychologised. From heart disease to endometriosis, countless women have endured years of invalidation before receiving accurate diagnoses. AI systems trained on such data inherit a skewed clinical worldview—one in which women's pain is under-recorded, misattributed, or systematically deprioritised. A symptom checker might suggest anxiety instead of a cardiac event because that is what the data historically shows. Not because it is accurate, but because *women's pain was rarely written down in ways the system could learn from.*

The same holds for racialised patients. Numerous studies have shown that Black patients in the United States receive less pain medication than white patients for the same conditions. That disparity, encoded in medical records, is invisible to an algorithm unless explicitly corrected. If AI is trained on such records without scrutiny, it may come to "learn" that Black patients require less intervention. The system then becomes a new site of exclusion—not through malice, but through *the codification of omission*.

This pattern extends beyond individual symptoms to broader diagnostic frameworks. Consider autism spectrum disorder. For decades, diagnostic criteria were developed around male presentations of autism, particularly in young white boys. As a result, girls, women, and people of colour were routinely missed—often being diagnosed much later, or mislabelled with anxiety or behavioural disorders. When AI systems are trained on data reflecting this diagnostic bias, they internalise a distorted baseline of what autism "looks like." As a result, these tools may underperform precisely where diagnostic correction is most needed. They do not fix the silence; they *formalise it.*

Nor is this limited to diagnosis. AI-based triage tools, increasingly deployed in emergency departments and call centres, are also susceptible. These systems rely on symptom input and severity scoring to determine urgency. But what happens when a patient's symptom language does not match the model's expectations? A South Asian woman describing heaviness in her chest may not trigger the same urgency as a white man reporting "chest pain." A neurodivergent individual who struggles with verbal articulation may input vague or non-standard descriptions. The system, unless specifically trained to account for linguistic and cultural variance, may misclassify them as low-risk. *Their voice enters the system, but is rendered unintelligible.*

Such systems are rarely transparent in their failure. Unlike a human clinician who might recognise misunderstanding and ask clarifying questions, an algorithm simply scores, categorises, and outputs a recommendation. If the model fails to capture the meaning behind a patient's words, it does not acknowledge uncertainty; it *continues confidently in error.* This unearned certainty can be particularly dangerous for marginalised patients, who may already face institutional distrust and scepticism. When the system dismisses them, they are left without recourse—misheard by a mechanism that cannot explain its decisions.

There is also a more insidious dynamic at play: *the illusion of inclusion.* Healthcare systems may deploy AI under the premise of expanding access or removing human bias. But if the underlying data and design choices are not critically interrogated, these tools may serve to automate exclusion more efficiently. This is especially dangerous because algorithmic decisions often carry an aura of objectivity. Patients who are deprioritised by a triage tool may not even realise that a computational model made that call—or that their symptoms were ignored not due to malice, but due to absence in the training set.

The marginalisation perpetuated by these systems is rarely intentional, but that does not make it any less harmful. In fact, it is precisely the *unintentionality*—the passive reproduction of bias through technical systems—that makes it harder to detect and challenge. Silence becomes harder to name when it is hidden inside statistical outputs. Who is responsible when a system consistently overlooks the needs of transgender patients because its training data includes no trans individuals? Who is accountable when a model fails to flag symptoms of lupus in Black women because they were historically underdiagnosed? *When voice is missing from data, injustice becomes procedural.*

Some developers have begun to recognise these limitations, working to diversify training datasets or introduce fairness audits. But the challenge goes deeper than inclusion. *It is about epistemology—what counts as knowledge in the system.* AI does not just need more data from marginalised groups; it needs to learn to *listen differently*. Clinical intuition often emerges from narrative, from the patient's story and how it unfolds over time. Algorithms, by contrast, reduce complexity into features and probabilities. They favour signals that are quantifiable, repeatable, and legible within the model's architecture. Much of what matters in human experience—ambivalence, ambiguity, cultural nuance—is filtered out in the preprocessing stage. The cost of this filtration is the erasure of difference.

One illustrative case comes from natural language processing tools used in mental health triage. Several startups have developed chatbots to assess suicide risk based on text input. But these systems often struggle with dialect, irony, and culturally specific expressions of distress. A Black teenager using vernacular or indirect references to depression may not trigger the same alerts as a white peer expressing sadness in more clinically expected terms. The algorithm does not decode meaning; it scans for keywords. Without culturally competent design, *it cannot hear pain spoken in unfamiliar tongues.*

To build systems that do not reinforce silence, we must move beyond the narrow frame of technical performance. It is not enough for an algorithm to be "accurate" on average. It must be just, interpretable, and sensitive to *which voices it privileges and which it erases.* This demands structural shifts—not only in how data is collected, but in who defines what counts as relevant information, whose experiences shape the model, and how dissent is accommodated.

Listening, in medicine as in life, is not a passive act. It is a form of recognition. When AI systems fail to hear marginalised voices, they are not just making bad predictions; they are reproducing a history of epistemic injustice—of deciding whose experience counts and whose can be ignored. This is not a computational problem. It is a cultural and political one.

The question is not whether AI can be trained to hear everyone equally. The question is whether we, as a society, are willing to confront the hierarchies that determine who gets to speak in the first place. If we build systems atop those hierarchies, we cannot expect them to dismantle what they were designed to ignore. We must build differently—starting not from the data we have, but from *the voices we have yet to listen to.*

Narrative Medicine vs. Predictive Models

A pulse can be measured. A lab result can be plotted. But when a patient says, "Something doesn't feel right," they are offering something else entirely—something harder to quantify, yet often more clinically significant than any metric. This is the domain of narrative medicine: the practice of attending to the stories people tell about their bodies, their suffering, their hopes, and their fears. It is a form of diagnostic listening rooted in the idea that *meaning*—not just data—drives healing. Predictive models, by contrast, are trained to strip away meaning in favour of pattern recognition. They are built not to hear stories, but to extract signals. That distinction is not merely methodological—it is philosophical. It raises urgent questions about what counts as knowledge in modern medicine, and what is lost when listening is outsourced to machines.

The core promise of predictive modelling in healthcare is efficiency. By analysing vast quantities of data—electronic health records, wearable sensor streams, imaging datasets, genetic profiles—AI systems can flag risks, suggest diagnoses, and recommend interventions with speed and scale previously unthinkable. But the very architecture of these systems demands that experience be encoded in discrete, numerical inputs. *Stories are not data-friendly.* They are messy, nonlinear, and context-dependent. Their power lies in their texture and unpredictability—in the parts that do not fit the template. In transforming medicine into a computational problem, predictive systems favour the legible over the lived.

The contrast becomes starkest in the clinic. A physician trained in narrative medicine may spend the first ten minutes of a consultation listening—*really* listening—to how a patient describes their symptoms, how they make sense of their illness, how it connects to the rhythms of their life. They may note pauses, emotion, metaphors, inconsistencies. This attention is not peripheral; it is diagnostic. A patient who describes "a heaviness, like I'm walking through water" might be conveying the early signs of depression, even if they never use that word. A patient with diabetes who says, "I stopped checking my blood sugar after my mum died," is revealing a psychological context essential to understanding adherence. Predictive models, by contrast, reduce this complexity to structured fields: ICD codes, blood glucose levels, medication refill histories. The story collapses into variables.

Some defenders of AI argue that this is not a flaw but a feature. After all, narrative is inherently subjective, prone to bias, and difficult to standardise. Stories vary based on language, culture, memory, and education. They are often contradictory or incomplete. Predictive systems promise to correct for this by anchoring decision-making in empirical regularities. But this appeal to objectivity is misleading. *All data is theory-laden.* What gets measured, how it is labelled, and which outcomes are prioritised are all shaped by human judgement. A system that predicts "non-adherence risk" based on refill history may inadvertently penalise patients with unstable housing or undocumented status. A model that flags "high-cost patients" may conflate clinical complexity with systemic disadvantage. Without the interpretive frame that narrative provides, these outputs risk becoming detached from reality.

Consider the case of a middle-aged man hospitalised three times in six months for uncontrolled hypertension. A predictive tool might label him a high-utiliser and recommend care coordination. But a physician practising narrative medicine might discover that the patient lost his job and housing after caring for a dying spouse, and has been rationing medications while sleeping in his car. The prediction is not wrong—but *it is incomplete.* The real insight comes not from the model's output, but from the story that explains *why* the output exists. Without that layer of meaning, even accurate predictions can mislead.

This divergence has ethical implications as well. Predictive systems are not neutral observers; they shape the clinical agenda. If a model predicts low likelihood of benefit from a treatment, it may never be offered. If it assigns a patient low risk, symptoms may be dismissed. This is not hypothetical. In 2019, a widely used algorithm in the United States was found to systematically underestimate the health needs of Black patients because it used healthcare spending as a proxy for health status. Black patients, who historically receive less care, were coded as lower risk—not because they were healthier, but because *they had less access to care.* Here, the predictive model overruled the possibility of a different story. The result was not merely a misclassification; it was a *systematic silencing.*

Narrative medicine resists this silencing by foregrounding the patient's voice. It insists that meaning cannot be outsourced. The practice emerged in part as a response to the growing mechanisation of medicine—the sense that the patient had become invisible behind a wall of scans, lab reports, and checklists. It argues that healing begins not with data extraction, but with *recognition*: the moment when a clinician sees the patient not just as a case, but as a person. That act of recognition is relational, not computational. It cannot be automated.

Yet this is not an argument for rejecting technology. Predictive models can be extraordinarily useful—particularly in surfacing hidden patterns, triaging scarce resources, and anticipating deterioration before it becomes visible. The question is not whether to use them, but *how*. At their best, predictive tools should augment clinical judgment, not replace it. They should inform—but never dictate—the conversation between patient and provider. When models are treated as definitive, they occlude the very uncertainty that makes medicine humane. When they are used reflexively, they foreclose the possibility of a story that does not fit.

There is also a deeper epistemological tension at work. Narrative medicine treats illness as a *situated experience*—something lived, interpreted, and given meaning within a social and cultural world. Predictive models treat illness as a *statistical deviation*—something detectable through deviation from normative patterns. Both approaches seek understanding, but they arrive at different kinds of truth. The former asks: "What is this person going through?" The latter asks: "What does this data point suggest?" In the gap between these questions lies a growing fault line in contemporary healthcare.

Reckoning with this divide requires more than integrating narrative notes into EHRs or adding "patient voice" tokens to model training. It demands a cultural shift in what we value as evidence. Medical training must not only teach clinicians how to interpret data, but how to *listen well*. Health systems must make time and space for storytelling—not as an indulgence, but as a core clinical competency. Technologists must design systems that can accommodate ambiguity, contradiction, and non-standard expressions. And patients must be treated not as data sources, but as narrators of their own experience.

There are signs of progress. Some institutions are experimenting with hybrid models that combine statistical prediction with narrative elicitation. Others are embedding medical anthropologists or narrative consultants into care teams. But the pace is slow, and the pressure to automate is strong. In a system that rewards throughput and quantifiable outcomes, storytelling can feel like a luxury. That is precisely why it must be defended.

Narrative medicine and predictive models are not mutually exclusive. But they are grounded in different assumptions about what it means to know, to care, and to act. As AI becomes more entrenched in clinical decision-making, we must be vigilant about what is being lost—not just in terms of accuracy, but in terms of *relationship*. A model may predict that a patient is unlikely to benefit from further intervention. A narrative may reveal that what the patient wants most is not a cure, but to be understood. Only one of these paths begins by asking: *What matters to you?*

The future of medicine will not be decided solely by advances in computation. It will be shaped by whether we remember that health is not just about outcomes, but about *meaning*. In the rush to predict, we must not forget to listen. Stories do not fit neatly into algorithms, but they remain medicine's oldest, and often most powerful, diagnostic tool. We abandon them at our peril.

Case Study: A Misread Life

The algorithm predicted stability. The clinical dashboard showed green. But the patient was not fine—she was deteriorating in plain sight, and no one noticed until it was too late. This is not a cautionary tale from the future. It is a case study grounded in the present, where well-intentioned automation overrode clinical intuition, flattening a complex human life into a risk score that quietly misled everyone in the room.

Amira was a 63-year-old woman living with multiple chronic conditions: type 2 diabetes, hypertension, and mild cognitive impairment. She had been managing her health relatively independently, aided by a home health monitoring programme that tracked her glucose levels, blood pressure, weight, and step count through a suite of connected devices. Her clinicians relied on a predictive analytics platform integrated into the hospital's electronic health record system—a model designed to flag patients at risk of hospital readmission within 30 days, using hundreds of variables drawn from previous admissions, demographics, biometric data, and medication adherence logs.

For six weeks, Amira's data told a story of control. Her glucose readings hovered in the high-normal range. Her blood pressure was slightly elevated but consistent. She took her medications with regularity. The AI system assigned her a "low-risk" status with high confidence. Her clinician, already managing a panel of nearly 2,000 patients, noted the green status and deprioritised a follow-up. The case was invisible—functionally triaged out of attention.

What no system detected was what Amira's daughter later described as "the quiet collapse." A normally gregarious woman, Amira had stopped attending her local senior centre, no longer answered phone calls, and had recently complained to a neighbour that "nothing tastes right anymore." Her sensor data remained steady, but she had started skipping meals. Her weight dropped slightly—within range—but not enough to trigger an alert. Her step count decreased, but only modestly, and the machine learning model interpreted the dip as age-related variability, not an early sign of physical and emotional decline.

When Amira was finally brought to the hospital by ambulance—after being found semi-conscious on her sofa—she was diagnosed with acute kidney injury, dehydration, and signs of undiagnosed depression. Her sodium levels were dangerously high, a consequence of erratic fluid intake. The clinicians were shocked. The system had not just missed the deterioration; it had insisted on her wellness. The green flag had given everyone a false sense of reassurance.

This was not a failure of signal, but of interpretation. *The model did what it was trained to do.* It used historical and biometric data to estimate the likelihood of readmission—a statistical abstraction. It did not, and could not, ask whether Amira had withdrawn from her social routine, whether she had lost interest in eating, or whether the nuances of her facial affect suggested loneliness, fear, or confusion. These were not features in the training data. They were parts of a narrative that lived outside the algorithm's reach.

The clinician, pressed for time and inundated with dashboards, deferred to the system's assessment. The automation bias was subtle but powerful: the model appeared objective, mathematically precise, and free of human error. But its output lacked context. The probability score supplanted a deeper question—*what is happening in this person's life?* Amira became her metrics.

This case illustrates a growing concern in modern medicine: that clinical decision-making is increasingly shaped by systems designed to simplify, compress, and prioritise. In high-volume settings, automation offers relief—a way to manage overwhelming complexity with quantitative clarity. But when that simplification becomes a proxy for judgment, systems that were meant to assist can start to dominate.

It would be easy to interpret Amira's story as a one-off failure of a flawed system. But the problem is more systemic. Predictive models are trained on historical data, which reflect the biases, omissions, and constraints of the health system itself. These models optimise for outcomes that are legible—readmission, mortality, cost—not necessarily meaningful to patients. They do not "see" the lived experience between appointments. And because models are designed to detect correlations, not causation, they often cannot explain *why* a patient is changing—only that a change statistically matters or doesn't.

Amira's decline was slow, multidimensional, and deeply human. Her mild cognitive impairment made it difficult for her to articulate the change she was experiencing. Her pride prevented her from reaching out. Her cultural background—North African, widowed, living alone in a suburban area with limited mobility—meant she was socially isolated, and reluctant to bother her overburdened doctor. These layers of context did not enter the model. The risk score reflected her data; it did not reflect her.

One might argue that the clinician should have intervened regardless of the model's output. But this, too, misrepresents the realities of clinical work. In under-resourced systems, physicians are expected to make quick decisions across vast patient rosters, relying on prioritisation tools to surface concern. When those tools fail silently, the consequences are distributed—slow-moving, difficult to trace, and devastating.

There is a deeper ethical tension here. When a model recommends inaction, and harm follows, who is responsible? The clinician who deferred to the system? The developer who trained the model on incomplete features? The institution that prioritised efficiency over attention? Responsibility, in these scenarios, becomes dispersed—*conveniently unlocatable*. The system speaks with authority, but it is not accountable. And in that void, patients like Amira fall through the cracks.

More importantly, the presence of automation can erode the clinician's trust in their own judgment. In earlier years, Amira's doctor might have noticed something in her voice, her affect, or her story—a subtle cue that warranted a call or home visit. But with a model declaring "low risk," that intuition becomes suspect, an inefficiency in a system optimised for precision. The clinician begins to internalise the idea that care is best when standardised, even if that means overriding human concern.

What might have changed the outcome for Amira? Not better data alone. Her device streams were relatively complete. Not more alerts—those already contribute to alarm fatigue. What she needed was an interpretive layer between data and action: *someone to ask why the green light didn't feel right*. This does not require rejecting automation but rethinking its role. Rather than replacing clinical judgment, predictive systems should be *interrogated* by it. A green risk score should not be a signal to ignore, but a prompt to ask: "Is this right?"

The case also points to a structural need for more narrative integration. Technologies that track social engagement, emotional expression, or daily routine—when designed ethically and interpreted thoughtfully—could provide richer context. But even the best sensors cannot replace conversation. The question is not how to quantify Amira's life more thoroughly, but how to *honour its complexity*. This means making room in the clinical encounter for unstructured, unscripted narratives, and training systems to support—not silence—those stories.

Amira recovered physically, but not entirely. She was discharged into a care facility and never returned to her home.

Her daughter, when interviewed by the hospital's quality review board, said something that has stayed with many who read the report: *"Everything was working, but no one was listening."* It is a statement that should unsettle us—not because it indicts technology, but because it reveals our growing willingness to let systems do the listening for us.

This is not a rejection of predictive modelling. It is a call for humility. Systems can model patterns, but they cannot model lives. They can surface risk, but not meaning. And when they appear to know too much, they can quietly prevent us from asking the very questions that define medicine's purpose: *What matters to this person? What are they going through? What are we missing?* A misread life is not a data error. It is a moral failure—a failure to care.

Chapter 5
The Quantified Self and the Dissolving Patient

There was a time when health was something one *felt*—a sense of fatigue, vitality, malaise, or equilibrium—rather than a collection of digits blinking on a screen. Today, many wake not to the sensations of their bodies, but to dashboards: a sleep score of 78, a readiness index at 63, resting heart rate four beats higher than yesterday. Each number signals a call to action. For countless people, the very first moment of consciousness has already become clinical.

This chapter begins with a paradox: never before have individuals had such access to precise physiological information, yet never has certainty about one's own health been so elusive. The act of measurement, far from clarifying, often destabilises. The "quantified self"—a person reduced to streams of continuous data—embodies both the promise and the dilemma of contemporary medicine. As health becomes intelligible to machines, the person behind the metrics risks fading into obscurity.

Self-tracking technologies arrived under the banner of empowerment. The story was compelling: data would liberate users from ignorance, make care proactive, and render prevention personal. Indeed, in certain clinical contexts, these tools deliver precisely that. A diabetic, armed with a continuous glucose monitor, can act on minute-by-minute trends; a cardiac patient may avert an emergency thanks to real-time rhythm alerts. The technology itself is not the problem. It is the ubiquity, the normalization, the shift from *aid* to *identity* that raises urgent questions: when monitoring becomes selfhood, what is lost?

The act of observing, once episodic and professionalised, is now ambient and relentless. Steps, sleep, stress, calories, heart-rate variability, ovulation, mood, cognition—almost no domain remains untracked. Everyday life becomes a site of medical vigilance. A skipped workout is flagged as an event; a restless night triggers caution. The body is no longer trusted to speak; it must submit its testimony through quantification.

This shift carries cultural weight. The wearable transforms into a badge of discipline, proof of self-optimisation and responsibility. Yet what validates control simultaneously breeds anxiety. When every heartbeat is scored, every fluctuation is suspect. Metrics do not simply reflect reality—they begin to constitute it. You are not just measured; you become the measure.

The psychological consequences are subtle but profound. Waking to a "poor" recovery score can leave a person feeling depleted before even rising. Hormonal tracking may recast normal mood swings as pathology. The self becomes predictive rather than lived—a forecast, not a sensation. Health is no longer experienced; it is continuously evaluated.

Ironically, these tools often destabilise the very baselines they claim to define. Norms vary across platforms, from day to day, app to app. Proprietary algorithms obscure how targets are set. Users may hit one benchmark and fail another without understanding why. Health becomes a game with invisible rules, no referee in sight.

For those managing chronic illness, the disorientation is acute. A hypertensive patient may see consistent readings dismissed as "controlled" by one device, flagged as warning signs by another. Someone in remission from cancer may struggle to interpret fatigue or appetite changes through a tracker incapable of context. The pursuit of agency via data can easily flip into dependence, where well-being is mediated through sensor updates, algorithmic drift, and shifting thresholds.

More insidiously, the logic of care merges with the logic of control. Personalisation may appear patient-centred, but constant monitoring invites intervention in everyday behaviour. Diet, sleep, movement, mood—each becomes a calculated risk. One is no longer merely cared for; one is managed.

Consider a workplace wellness programme that adjusts insurance premiums based on wearable compliance, or an insurer reducing rewards when step counts fall short, irrespective of individual circumstances. Across the globe, the quantified self is less a participant and more a monitored subject—optimised, nudged, disciplined.

Framed as choice, this surveillance often leaves voluntariness hollow. Declining tracking can carry social or financial penalties. Even in theory, opting out may mark one as careless or resistant. The refusal to quantify becomes a moral judgement.

Who defines health, meanwhile, is rarely neutral. App developers and device manufacturers shape feedback loops with commercial imperatives. Notifications, gamified streaks, nudges—they are engineered not merely to inform, but to engage, to bind users to the system. What is presented as empowerment is often anxiety by design. Users believe they are in control; in truth, the system orchestrates the cues, sets the stakes, and judges the outcomes.

Continuous evaluation, opaque standards, and interpretive burden create subtle but chronic vigilance. What begins as insight can metastasise into stress. Fluctuations are endlessly interrogated: early warning or random noise? Users learn to anticipate, correct, optimise—sometimes at the expense of simply being.

Cultural and structural biases compound the problem. Predictive models are built on data from populations that are typically young, affluent, technologically fluent, and predominantly white. Those outside these norms—marginalised groups, those with atypical rhythms—may appear aberrant, their resilience misread as risk. Personalised care, in such cases, becomes a system of conformity: visibility and validation only for those who fit the model's template.

And yet, self-tracking cannot be dismissed wholesale. For some, wearables provide early warnings, structure, and validation otherwise absent. In communities with limited access to traditional care, they can offer a measure of autonomy. The question is not technology itself, but the ideology it carries: that life is most intelligible through measurement, that the self exists primarily as data, and that only the measurable is meaningful.

If health is reduced to numbers, what of the unquantifiable—grief, joy, intuition, doubt? These cannot be smoothed into dashboards, yet they are integral to the human experience. Most devices remain indifferent to these subtleties. Their failure is not error but omission—they simply do not listen.

As predictive care, continuous monitoring, and algorithmic nudges proliferate, we must ask: what kind of person is being shaped by these tools? Not simply what they measure, but what they teach users to value, to prioritise, to fear. The quantified self is an ideology, one that risks replacing wisdom with metrics, and human experience with the performance of control.

This chapter, then, is a defence of the human. It questions what is surrendered when identity is defined by dashboards. It is a reminder that care extends beyond metrics: it preserves meaning, narrative, and autonomy. And it invites us to reimagine health not as something endlessly tracked, but as something lived—messily, unpredictably, and freely.

When Monitoring Becomes Identity

Before the first cup of coffee is poured, before a single conscious decision is made, millions of people around the world check their health. But they do not consult a doctor, nor do they scan their own bodies in any intuitive sense. Instead, they glance at an app, a watch, or a wearable ring—checking a readiness score, a sleep quality index, or a heart rate variability graph. Increasingly, we do not just track our health. *We become what we track.*

This seemingly benign shift—subtle, incremental, and marketed as empowerment—has redefined what it means to be healthy or at risk. Where health was once an embodied state, a felt experience modulated by context and self-awareness, it is now rendered in constant streams of biometric data. Blood oxygen levels, movement trends, stress indices, recovery cycles: all updated in real time, with colour-coded guidance to match. But beneath the polished interfaces and chirpy nudges lies a conceptual overhaul of identity itself. To be a person in the age of self-tracking is, in part, to be a score.

The promise was alluring: know yourself better, act sooner, live longer. The first wave of consumer health tech sold itself on prevention through self-awareness. Fitbit's early advertisements featured empowered users "taking control" of their day, step by step. Later, more advanced platforms offered metrics previously confined to clinical settings—electrodermal activity, atrial fibrillation alerts, sleep phase analysis—delivered effortlessly to one's phone. On the surface, this seems like undeniable progress. But the deeper effect is epistemological. *Data becomes not just a tool for knowing health—it becomes health itself.*

The metrics do not merely reflect how we feel; they increasingly dictate how we interpret ourselves. A person who wakes up energised but sees a poor sleep score may question their own perception. Another who feels lethargic may find solace in a "green zone" readiness metric, assuming that fatigue is a misreading rather than a real cue. In this way, *biofeedback displaces self-trust*. Over time, the body's intuitive signals are overwritten by algorithmic interpretations, subtly reorganising whose voice counts in defining experience.

This shift has a particular resonance in a culture obsessed with optimisation. Once relegated to elite athletes and quantified self enthusiasts, performance tracking has gone mainstream. Productivity gurus, lifestyle influencers, and wellness platforms champion a form of health that is not merely functional but maximised. The ideal self is not just illness-free—it is always improving, always monitoring, always refining. Health is no longer a state to inhabit but a metric to pursue.

But in the pursuit of measurable perfection, people can become estranged from their own embodied realities. The idea of being "at risk" expands. A few nights of poor sleep, a decline in heart rate variability, or a deviation from trend lines can be interpreted not as variability but as vulnerability. *The concept of risk shifts from a probability to a daily identity.* You are not just someone with potential for illness—you are someone whose metrics suggest you might be failing at health.

This reframing has emotional consequences. Research on the psychological impact of self-tracking consistently shows a correlation between excessive monitoring and increased anxiety, particularly in those without clinical need. The constant inflow of data can foster a low-level vigilance, a hyperawareness of the body that borders on obsession. Instead of creating peace of mind, these tools often deliver a relentless subtext: *you are not quite right—yet.*

For individuals with health anxiety or perfectionistic tendencies, this can be corrosive. Rather than facilitating empowerment, devices become mechanisms of self-surveillance and guilt. Skipped steps, erratic sleep, or inconsistent biometrics are not simply deviations; they are moral failings. Even users who consciously resist these narratives often find themselves subtly influenced. The red zone feels like a reprimand, the green zone like a reward. Algorithms whisper approval or disappointment beneath every data point.

Moreover, the metrics themselves are not neutral. They are shaped by developers' assumptions about what constitutes "healthy," "optimal," or "normal." These definitions may not align with the lived experiences of users, particularly those outside the data sets on which the algorithms were trained. A person with atypical sleep cycles, a disability, or a chronic condition may find their metrics consistently framed as deficient—even when they feel stable and functional. *In such cases, self-tracking does not just fail to reflect the person; it actively misrepresents them.*

The psychological burden of this misalignment is often under-acknowledged. When the numbers suggest you are failing but your body says otherwise, who do you believe? When your experience is dismissed by an interface designed without your profile in mind, how do you reclaim agency? And when friends or clinicians treat your metrics as more authoritative than your words, what happens to your voice?

This conflict is not merely theoretical. Consider the rise of "data-based decisions" in clinical settings. A patient presents with fatigue and palpitations but their wearables show nothing alarming. A doctor, already overburdened, may deprioritise their account in favour of machine-readable evidence. Here, *monitoring technologies become gatekeepers of legitimacy*. If the system cannot see your suffering, it may not believe you are suffering.

Yet, for all its limitations, the data still matters. It can offer early warnings, identify patterns, support behavioural change.

The problem is not measurement—it is the conflation of measurement with meaning. Metrics can be useful cues; they are poor definitions of identity. When users begin to self-identify with their trends—when they feel "better" or "worse" purely based on their dashboard—we enter dangerous terrain. *Health becomes performative, lived in metrics, and filtered through a lens of constant self-appraisal.*

This performativity is reinforced by social structures. Apps that encourage sharing metrics, comparing scores, and maintaining streaks introduce an element of surveillance capitalism into the most intimate domains of life. You are not only tracking yourself—you are being tracked, categorised, and benchmarked against others. Social dashboards, health competitions, and incentivised programmes turn self-care into spectacle. The self becomes both the performer and the performed.

The result is a kind of bio-narcissism: a persistent preoccupation with one's internal state, interpreted not through felt sense but through feedback loops. Like staring into a digital mirror, users seek affirmation from metrics instead of meaning from experience. But a life lived in reference to numbers can begin to feel hollow. The spontaneous, the intuitive, the unmeasured—all risk being discounted.

In the long term, this redefinition of identity carries cultural consequences. If health is measured only by what can be tracked, then aspects of humanity that resist quantification—resilience, intuition, emotional richness—are devalued. People who thrive without optimisation may be seen as outliers, or worse, negligent. Meanwhile, those whose identities are overrun by biofeedback may find it increasingly difficult to differentiate between themselves and their scores.

The core tension is this: *we are using tools of surveillance to pursue a feeling of agency.* But surveillance and autonomy make uneasy companions. Monitoring may inform us, but when it begins to define us, we risk becoming prisoners of our own data. A healthy identity cannot be sustained through metrics alone. It requires space for ambiguity, room for self-trust, and the right to exist outside the logic of optimisation.

As this chapter will continue to explore, the quantified self is not just a technical evolution—it is a philosophical shift. It demands that we reconsider not only how we define health, but how we define the self. And as we navigate the world of predictive models, ambient surveillance, and algorithmic nudges, we must ask: *Who are we becoming when the data is always watching?*

Medicalization of Everyday Life

A person yawns mid-afternoon and glances at their wearable. "Recovery zone: orange. Energy forecast: moderate. Sleep debt: 74 minutes." With a quick swipe, they scroll through their hydration trends and receive a subtle suggestion to reduce caffeine after midday. No illness has been diagnosed, no complaint voiced. And yet, they find themselves adjusting behaviours under the influence of an ever-expanding digital regime of health oversight. *This is not medicine as response—it is medicine as presence.*

What was once the domain of the clinical—diagnosis, treatment, prognosis—has seeped into the textures of ordinary living. Eating, sleeping, walking, socialising, even feeling distracted at work—activities once seen as human variability or lifestyle choices—are now medicalised through personalised metrics, behavioural nudges, and risk stratification engines. Under the banner of "preventive care," health systems and tech platforms alike have begun to cast a wider net over everyday life, transforming the normal into the surveilled and the surveilled into the pathologised.

The concept of medicalisation is not new. Sociologists such as Ivan Illich and Peter Conrad have long argued that the boundaries of medicine expand as more aspects of life are interpreted through a biomedical lens. But today's iteration is not driven solely by doctors or healthcare systems—it is powered by algorithms, personalisation engines, and real-time data collection. What makes this moment distinct is not the expansion of medicine per se, but its *invisibility*. Care has become ambient. Oversight has become proactive. Intervention has become habitual.

Personalisation plays a central role in this shift. The promise of tailoring health advice to the individual—long a theoretical ideal—is now technologically feasible. With granular data about heart rate, glucose levels, sleep cycles, and even emotional tone (via voice analysis or typing speed), systems can deliver interventions that feel intimate, precise, and timely. But such intimacy masks a structural concern: *personalisation is often less about individual understanding and more about continuous optimisation against population norms.*

This is where the logic begins to blur. When a system tells you your glucose spike is "outside optimal range," it implies a deviation from an ideal—yet that ideal is often based on aggregated data, not your own history or context. When your smartwatch flags sedentary behaviour after 45 minutes of stillness, it is enforcing a movement pattern abstracted from generalised health recommendations. Even when accurate, these nudges are not neutral. They carry normative weight. *They suggest not only how you are, but how you ought to be.*

Over time, these repeated micro-interventions shift the psychological framing of behaviour. Choosing not to stand becomes an act of noncompliance. Eating a second helping turns into "risk exposure." Skipping a workout is not simply rest—it is a data point indicating backslide. What was once self-regulation becomes algorithmic governance, where the lines between lifestyle and treatment begin to dissolve. A person need not be ill to be treated as if they are perpetually at risk.

This risk-based framing is particularly insidious. Traditional medicine treated risk as a function of probability—useful, but separate from identity. Predictive systems, however, do not distinguish between current illness and future potential. A user may be flagged as "high risk" for type 2 diabetes or cardiovascular events based on behavioural indicators, family history, or minor biomarkers. These flags often lead to lifestyle prescriptions—adjust your diet, increase activity, reduce screen time—not as advice, but as *clinical directives.* And when non-compliance is logged, the system records not just behaviour, but deviation. *Risk becomes the default identity, with health defined as an ongoing act of conformity.*

This has cultural consequences. In environments where data-driven wellness is valorised—corporate wellness programmes, insurance platforms, elite health communities—non-participation can signal irresponsibility. A person who declines to monitor their metrics, who eats unpredictably or prefers rest over output, is not simply opting out. They are framed, subtly or overtly, as neglecting their health. *The choice to live unmeasured becomes a deviant stance.* This, in turn, reinforces a silent coercion: participate or be pathologised.

Further, the growing entanglement of healthcare and everyday behaviour raises questions of *jurisdiction.* Who has the authority to define what is healthy, and on what grounds? Should an app designer, a data scientist, or an actuarial model determine the thresholds that shape users' daily decisions? And when such determinations are baked into interfaces—prompting "smart" suggestions or shaping default choices—do users retain meaningful consent?

Consider the proliferation of digital wellness tools offered through employers. These platforms often reward engagement with lower insurance premiums, access to bonuses, or gamified recognition. But they also introduce surveillance into the private sphere under the guise of wellness. A step count may seem innocuous until it becomes a benchmark. A mood tracker may offer insights until it becomes an arbiter of performance. Here, *personalisation morphs into productivity infrastructure*, and care becomes a system of behavioural compliance.

Moreover, the scope of what is medicalised continues to widen. Loneliness, distraction, lack of focus, minor digestive fluctuations—all increasingly framed as health issues requiring digital solutions. While each of these can correlate with medical conditions, they are also part of ordinary life. When ordinary fluctuations are labelled as clinical risks, we lose the capacity to tolerate discomfort or accept ambiguity. We become patients not because we are unwell, but because the system cannot distinguish variability from vulnerability.

This erosion of the normal has psychological costs. People begin to interpret themselves as perpetually on the edge—of illness, of burnout, of decline. This mindset fosters what some psychologists call *anticipatory anxiety*—a low-grade vigilance born not from symptoms, but from the expectation of deterioration. And when systems flag risk but cannot guarantee outcomes, users are left in a state of unresolvable alertness. Always adjusting, never arriving.

Paradoxically, this expansion of medical oversight does not necessarily yield greater trust in health systems. As more aspects of life are drawn into the clinical domain, the threshold for meaningful attention rises. When every moment is monitored, the urgency of any particular alert diminishes. When every deviation is a risk, no risk feels actionable. This leads to *clinical fatigue*—a quiet scepticism or burnout among users who are overwhelmed by the constancy of care.

The medicalisation of everyday life also alters the patient-clinician relationship. Increasingly, patients arrive at appointments already carrying a quantified portrait of themselves—data from wearables, food logs, mood diaries. While such information can enhance diagnosis, it can also shift authority. Clinicians may feel pressure to validate or refute self-generated data, while patients may trust their metrics more than their practitioners. This dynamic reframes care as a negotiation between embodied experience and quantified evidence, with potential friction on both sides.

Some may argue that this is a net gain—more awareness, earlier interventions, better outcomes. But this optimism must be tempered with clarity about trade-offs. When data replaces dialogue, when risk replaces rest, and when optimisation becomes moralised, we edge towards a healthcare paradigm that is less about *being well* and more about *performing wellness*. In such a paradigm, care becomes control—and the patient becomes a project.

This is not an argument against technology or prevention. Rather, it is a call for vigilance in how we frame, deploy, and inhabit health systems that operate continuously. We must ask not only what these systems can measure, but what they *assume*. Not only what they predict, but what they *prioritise*. And not only whom they serve, but whom they silence.

To safeguard autonomy in this new terrain, we must preserve the distinction between *support* and *surveillance*, between *personalisation* and *prescription*. That boundary—often soft, often shifting—is where freedom resides. It is the space in which people can be more than their metrics, and where care can be something we *choose*, not simply something we *comply with*.

Anxiety by Design

A user wakes at 6:30 a.m. and instinctively checks the small screen on their wrist before even getting out of bed. The device informs them their "readiness score" is suboptimal. Their sleep stages were imbalanced, heart rate variability trended lower than usual, and the system suggests a "low-stress day." But the calendar disagrees: a presentation, childcare logistics, and two deadlines loom. The physiological insight does not provide clarity—it introduces conflict. *Should they trust the body or the biometric?*

What masquerades as empowerment in many health technologies is often a form of anxiety dressed in interface design. The modern health app is not neutral. It does not merely reflect data; it frames it, qualifies it, and applies meaning—sometimes clinical, sometimes moral. In doing so, it subtly reframes the user's relationship to their body, not as lived experience but as a site of continuous performance evaluation. *Selfhood becomes an interface problem, and the solution is more feedback.*

This shift is neither accidental nor benign. App and wearable ecosystems are meticulously engineered to sustain user engagement. Design teams draw heavily from behavioural psychology and persuasive computing frameworks to ensure that users return repeatedly, interact regularly, and rely increasingly on the system's assessments. Metrics are colour-coded for affective immediacy: green for good, red for warning. Streaks gamify compliance. Notifications arrive with impeccable timing, not to inform, but to *nudge*. The interface becomes a therapist, a coach, and an examiner—simultaneously.

The result is a user not merely informed by their data, but *psychologically entangled with it*. When a sleep app notes elevated disturbance, many users retrospectively feel tired—even if they woke up feeling fine. When a stress score dips below baseline, users report irritability, even before experiencing any overt triggers. This feedback loop is not simply reactive—it is formative. It guides perception, not just behaviour. The quantified self becomes the *interpreted self*, shaped by readings it did not consciously produce and cannot fully contest.

It is important to understand the architecture of this dynamic. These systems rely on continuous biometric surveillance—heart rate, movement, temperature, respiration, sometimes even galvanic skin response or pulse oximetry. But the data are often noisy, imprecise, and context-deprived. To generate actionable outputs, the raw signals must be processed through statistical smoothing, normative modelling, and interpretative heuristics. That "readiness score" on your screen is not a direct reading—it is *an algorithmic opinion*. Yet the design conceals this uncertainty. The interface offers declarative certainty where the science is probabilistic at best.

Here lies the core tension: *users are given the illusion of self-knowledge, but they are actually engaging with system-generated narratives.* These narratives often frame the user as deficient, lagging, or non-compliant. The constant push to optimise sleep, stress, hydration, movement—under the guise of health promotion—can easily become a relentless moral project. Even rest must be efficient. Even calm must be logged. *Wellness becomes not a state of being, but a checklist to satisfy.*

While proponents argue that this level of feedback increases autonomy, it can just as easily undermine it. Users begin to second-guess intuition, defer to sensors, and outsource self-evaluation. They may avoid certain foods, abandon activities, or structure their day based on device guidance, even in the absence of symptoms or discomfort. What was once self-care becomes *self-surveillance*. Agency becomes reaction. And this dependency is not accidental—it is designed.

Market incentives reinforce this loop. Health tech companies benefit from high engagement and low attrition. More anxiety often means more usage, more check-ins, more subscription renewals. A user who obsessively monitors sleep metrics is more valuable than one who glances weekly. In this economy, *worry is profitable*. And so features are crafted not just to reassure, but to provoke—subtly, persistently. A red sleep score here, a falling heart rate trend there, a prompt to "take a mindful moment" even when no distress was felt. These cues generate ambient unease. Not enough to cause panic—just enough to keep the user *returning*.

Importantly, this anxiety is not evenly distributed. People already navigating chronic illness, mental health challenges, or disability may find themselves triangulating between symptoms and scores, sometimes with conflicting results. A person with generalised anxiety disorder might find that their biofeedback app confirms their worry rather than easing it. A woman with perimenopausal symptoms may be told her cycle data are "inconsistent," implying error where there is natural variability. In these moments, the interface does not empower—it *invalidates*.

The same holds true for marginalised groups. Algorithms trained predominantly on healthy, young, white male populations often misinterpret signals from others. For example, wearable heart rate sensors have been shown to have lower accuracy on darker skin tones due to the way optical sensors absorb light. If an app misreads your physiology but still issues authoritative guidance, it introduces not only error, but *epistemic harm*—a form of knowing that obscures rather than clarifies. And when the user blames themselves for "not doing it right," the system's authority remains intact.

There is also a subtle erosion of privacy within this engagement model. The more anxious the user, the more data they produce. That data becomes part of an ecosystem—sometimes encrypted and protected, but often commodified, aggregated, or sold. Even in anonymised form, it informs insurance models, advertising algorithms, employer wellness programmes. A user's elevated cortisol may translate not into personalised care, but into actuarial risk. The anxiety, it seems, flows both ways.

Yet the cultural narrative surrounding these technologies remains overwhelmingly positive. To critique health apps is often to be seen as anti-innovation or anti-empowerment. But recognising *the cost of empowerment* is not the same as rejecting it. It is an insistence that power, to be meaningful, must be transparent, contestable, and *optional*. When users feel unable to step away without fear of neglecting their health, that is not empowerment—it is captivity.

Designers, developers, and clinicians need to ask deeper questions. What constitutes a useful metric? Who defines the thresholds? What are the emotional consequences of being told, daily, that you are insufficiently recovered, under-hydrated, or overexerted? And how can systems support flourishing rather than compliance?

Some promising shifts are underway. A small number of platforms now allow users to customise their feedback—turning off scores, limiting notifications, or contextualising alerts with explanations. Others offer periodic "data sabbaticals" or encourage intuitive check-ins alongside metrics. These gestures are nascent, but important. They suggest that *healthy technology does not require constant visibility*. Sometimes, support means *stepping back*.

Ultimately, the goal is not to eliminate self-tracking, but to reframe its role. Data should *illuminate*, not dominate. Insight should *enrich*, not destabilise. And systems designed to care should not make people *feel worse* about being themselves.

Until then, users must tread carefully in these ambient diagnostic landscapes. Because in a world where the body is always being monitored, and the mind always being nudged, it is not health we optimise—it is obedience. And the cost of that obedience, when delivered through a cheerful interface, is often *a quiet, daily anxiety too normalised to notice.*

The Data-Driven Self as a Moving Target

In the analogue age, health was largely a binary matter: one felt well, or one did not. Diagnosis came with symptoms, and recovery was measured in the return of equilibrium. Today, the quantified body dissolves that clarity. With the proliferation of wearable devices, health platforms, and algorithmic baselining, individuals are no longer judged against general standards of wellbeing but against a personal profile of ever-evolving, system-defined metrics. What was once a shared map of biological norms has become a private labyrinth of shifting baselines, recalibrated risks, and interpretative volatility. *Health is no longer what you feel—it is what your data says you are becoming.*

This transformation is sold as precision. Instead of comparing patients against crude population averages, data-driven health promises a more accurate assessment by learning from each individual's unique physiology, rhythms, and patterns. In theory, a personalised norm is a better norm. A heart rate that appears elevated for the general public may be typical for a particular athlete. A sleep pattern that seems erratic might be ideal for someone with polyphasic tendencies. But the very concept of personal baselining introduces a paradox: if the "normal" is always recalculating, then the patient is forever being measured against a target that moves with them. *Stability gives way to flux. Clarity gives way to drift.*

Consider how this plays out in practice. A user wears a health-tracking device that monitors sleep efficiency. In the first month, the system gathers sufficient data to set a personal baseline. Over time, that baseline updates—perhaps because the user travels across time zones, becomes more active, changes their diet, or simply ages. The software quietly adapts. A score of 82% sleep efficiency might be "excellent" in January, "average" in May, and "poor" by October. The user has not changed; the frame has. The experience of wellbeing remains constant, but the narrative supplied by the system deteriorates. Anxiety follows. The problem isn't health decline—it's data drift.

This phenomenon is not limited to sleep metrics. Blood glucose monitors, menstrual cycle trackers, heart rate variability sensors, and stress detection tools all operate within adaptive thresholds. They learn and update. But these shifts often occur without explanation or interpretability. The user receives scores, alerts, or warnings without understanding the logic behind the system's changing thresholds. One week a "green zone" heart rate is 72 bpm. The next, it's 68. Why? Because the algorithm detected a trend. But trends are not truths. They are artefacts of computational smoothing, model fit, and noise filtration. *The body remains constant, but the system narrates variation.*

This constant recalibration creates a kind of epistemic vertigo for patients. If one's norm is always in motion, then what constitutes improvement? What justifies concern? Should a sudden deviation be taken seriously, or is it a false alarm born from an unstable baseline? Clinicians, too, are increasingly asked to interpret data dashboards with colour-coded trends and probabilistic risk scores that lack standardised thresholds. They are forced to triangulate between the patient's self-reported experience and the system's opaque signals. When the two diverge, it is not always obvious which voice to trust. The result is diagnostic dissonance.

For example, a patient managing long COVID may report improvement in energy and function, but their wearable shows declining readiness scores and increased variability in resting metrics. Is the patient in denial, or is the model misreading non-linear recovery? Another patient may be flagged as "pre-diabetic" based on micro-shifts in glucose variability, even though no diagnostic threshold has been crossed. These nudges—while well-intended—can create *anticipatory pathologisation*. The person becomes a patient before illness appears, simply because their trendline disagrees with their experience. In effect, *the self becomes suspicious by default.*

This issue becomes more acute when we consider how different platforms calculate and present "personalised" norms. One fitness app may use a 14-day rolling average. Another prefers a 30-day median filtered through activity class. Some systems rely on population-level comparisons first, then adjust based on user behaviour. Others reverse the order. The result is that the same person may receive conflicting assessments from two systems tracking the same physiology. One may declare "optimal performance," while another issues a warning. *The problem is not disagreement—it is incoherence*. When every system defines the target differently, the user loses their epistemic anchor.

And yet these platforms rarely acknowledge their own plasticity. Interface design tends to present outputs as stable, certain, and empirically grounded. The score appears definitive, the trend obvious, the alert justified. But underlying this presentation is a dynamic model architecture that is constantly retraining, re-weighting, and rebalancing itself. Few users are aware of this volatility. Fewer still are given the option to understand or challenge it. Personalised medicine, it turns out, can be deeply impersonal in its logic. The human subject is reduced to *the object of algorithmic interpretation*—informed, but not included.

There is also a deeper philosophical tension at play. Traditional medicine often operated with static diagnostic categories—hypertension, diabetes, major depression—grounded in observable thresholds or clinical criteria. The data-driven model, by contrast, emphasises gradients, probabilities, and continuous monitoring. It sees health not as a binary state but as a probabilistic landscape—one in which every data point is a clue and every deviation a potential signal. This can be helpful in early detection, but it can also be *destabilising*. The self becomes *a moving target in an uncertain game*, judged not by symptoms, but by deviation from a model whose logic is undisclosed.

The impact on patient psychology is significant. Studies have begun to show that users of continuous monitoring systems often report increased health anxiety, despite the absence of overt pathology. They experience a persistent sense of "not being quite right," driven not by feeling unwell, but by seeing red flags in their dashboard. This anxiety is compounded by the fact that these systems often fail to contextualise their findings. A rise in resting heart rate may be due to travel, caffeine, or a sleepless night—but the system flags it regardless, and the user is left to wonder. *Uncertainty becomes pathology. Data becomes doubt.*

Importantly, this issue is not a failure of personalisation per se. The problem lies in *how personalisation is implemented*—through adaptive models that lack transparency, communicate poorly, and often fail to explain their own logic. A truly empowering personalised system would offer interpretability: showing not just the score, but the confidence interval; not just the alert, but the reasoning. It would invite users to co-interpret their data, not just receive it. It would be a partner in health, not a diagnostician on a pedestal.

Moreover, the instability of personalised baselines poses challenges for longitudinal care. Imagine a patient being monitored over two years by a wearable that adjusts their norm every month. By the time a clinician examines the full history, the reference point may have changed dozens of times. Comparing current metrics to those from a year ago becomes meaningless if the baselines have evolved in the interim. Continuity of care, once grounded in stable reference points, is now filtered through *a kaleidoscope of algorithmic redefinitions*.

And yet, despite these concerns, the push towards adaptive personalisation continues—driven by market demand, data abundance, and the seductive logic of precision. What is missing is *critical design literacy*. We need systems that foreground not just what they know, but how they know it. We need interfaces that teach users how to interpret variability, recognise artefacts, and understand confidence margins. And we need clinical frameworks that bridge the gap between model-driven baselines and human experience. Otherwise, we risk creating a generation of patients who are perfectly tracked, thoroughly measured, and utterly confused.

In this unfolding landscape, the most pressing question is not whether personalised baselines are good or bad. It is: *Who controls the narrative of normality?* If that narrative is invisible, volatile, and proprietary, then even the most personalised system may fail to serve the person. Because clarity is not a function of precision alone—it is the result of coherence, dialogue, and trust. And without those, the data-driven self remains just that: a target in motion, forever seeking a centre it cannot find.

Chapter 6
The Clinician's Dilemma

The promise of artificial intelligence in medicine has long been framed as liberation: freeing clinicians from the tedium of administrative tasks, the guesswork of diagnosis, the limits of human attention. Yet, paradoxically, its integration may accomplish the opposite. As machine learning systems become fixtures in clinical practice, the physician's role shifts—not simply streamlined, but fundamentally redefined. The modern clinician is less an autonomous expert than a mediator, an operator, an interpreter of algorithmic outputs. AI does not merely offer a second opinion; it reshapes what it means to *have* a first one. And in doing so, it confronts practitioners with a dilemma that is no longer hypothetical: how does one practise medicine when human judgment must coexist with, defer to, or even justify itself against the machine?

At the core lies a subtle but profound shift in authority. For centuries, medical expertise rested on a cultivated interplay of training, intuition, pattern recognition, and interpersonal attunement. Diagnosis was as much art as science. But when predictive models begin to outperform humans in narrow domains—radiographic analysis, dermatology, early sepsis detection—the allure of machine precision can overshadow trust in human judgment. A probability score for pneumonia, a highlighted radiograph, or a saliency map no longer merely guides; it demands attention, sometimes compliance. Disagreeing with the system now requires defence.

These ripples extend far beyond the consultation. AI-generated recommendations are often logged in the medical record. Overriding an algorithm is no longer just a clinical decision; it is documented, reviewable, and potentially liable. Practitioners are compelled to weigh not only what is medically appropriate, but what is administratively defensible. The shift is subtle yet corrosive: discretion becomes conditional, exercised in the shadow of auditability. The clinician answers not only to the patient but also to the machine's logic.

Trust—both in AI and in oneself—becomes fraught. When does following a model constitute abdication of judgment? When does resisting it verge on negligence? Younger clinicians, trained in AI-integrated environments, may see the model as a natural extension of their toolkit. Experienced practitioners, however, may feel their hard-won craft quietly displaced. The tension is not merely generational; it is epistemological. It concerns who defines knowledge, and how.

Consider emergency triage, increasingly shaped by predictive analytics. Algorithms assist in decisions on admission, priority, and placement, trained on vast historical datasets, optimised for throughput and outcomes. Efficiency and consistency improve, but subtle cues—an anxious tone, a concerned relative, a fleeting expression of deterioration—remain unmeasured and unseen. What is not measured is invisible to the model.

Yet accountability remains human. Clinicians are responsible for outcomes, even when guided by systems they cannot interrogate. Most are neither trained to evaluate machine learning models, nor to assess bias in training data, nor to parse algorithmic uncertainty. And yet, they are expected to act as if the tools were transparent. A quiet epistemic coercion emerges: trust the system, even when comprehension is impossible, lest scepticism appear negligent.

The consequences are deeper still. AI often multiplies, rather than reduces, cognitive and administrative load. Documentation, alerts, decision points, data streams from wearables, portals, and ambient sensors all demand attention. Efficiency becomes a labyrinth of pings, audits, and automated noise. This digital burden increasingly drives clinician dissatisfaction and burnout, turning every action into a potential contribution to future optimisation. Physicians find themselves simultaneously caring for patients and training the very systems that might one day supplant them.

Even more concerning is the erosion of tacit knowledge. Clinical intuition—recognising atypical presentations, rare syndromes, or subtle interpersonal cues—is acquired through experience and difficult to codify. AI integration risks marginalising this wisdom. When practitioners rely on system outputs and are penalised for divergence, intuition atrophies. Medicine becomes procedural; care, compliance.

The ethical stakes are profound. Empathy, presence, and moral judgment—qualities central to healing—cannot be reduced to data. A reassuring touch, attentive listening, compassionate communication—these are forms of knowledge no algorithm can replicate. If training prioritises system fluency over these skills, the human core of medicine risks erosion.

Yet, rejecting AI entirely is neither feasible nor desirable. Its benefits are tangible: early detection of retinal disease, improved cancer screening, decision support in intensive care. Embracing these advances demands a new professionalism: one fluent in clinical reasoning *and* computational logic, capable of questioning the system while benefiting from it. The clinician of the future must be interpreter and interlocutor, able to follow, pause, and dissent judiciously.

This hybrid role necessitates changes in education, institutional culture, and ethics. Clinicians must learn to interrogate AI tools, understand biases and limitations, and practise critical oversight. Healthcare institutions must foster environments where questioning a model is safe, where disagreement is part of discourse rather than a liability.

Professional standards must evolve: judgment in the age of AI is not mere accuracy, but discernment.

Ultimately, the clinician's challenge is not man versus machine; it is the preservation of humanity within a system increasingly shaped by computational logic. Core values—trust, empathy, care—must endure, even as the tools of practice evolve. For patients, precision is insufficient; presence is irreplaceable. And presence, in its fullness, remains entirely human.

Between Expertise and Obsolescence

A radiologist working in a metropolitan hospital opens a scan on her monitor. Before she has a chance to form an impression, an automated label appears: "Likely pulmonary nodule, malignancy risk 83%." A soft chime sounds, and a box lights up with recommended next steps. She pauses. Her experience tells her the result may be a false positive. But to override the system, she will have to submit a justification, fill in a form, and potentially trigger a peer-review process. She clicks "Accept." Not because she believes the model is right, but because *it's easier to agree with the machine than to stand against it.* This is not an isolated case of convenience overriding confidence. It is a snapshot of the larger tectonic shift occurring in medicine: the slow reconfiguration of professional authority in the presence of machine intelligence.

Artificial intelligence is not merely altering clinical tools—it is altering the very terms of clinical expertise. In theory, AI augments the physician, offering sharper diagnostics, predictive insights, and data-driven precision. In practice, it can unsettle the clinician's role, provoke uncertainty, and shift accountability away from human discretion. The tension is not between "using AI" and "not using AI"—it is between *knowing* and *deferring to what the system says.* For many clinicians, this produces a persistent cognitive strain: *if the machine is more accurate, then what am I? And if I still matter, then when should I say no to the machine?*

Nowhere is this dilemma more visible than in specialties that depend heavily on pattern recognition—radiology, dermatology, pathology. In these fields, machine learning models are trained on massive image datasets to spot early-stage tumours, subtle lesions, or rare presentations with superhuman speed. In some trials, their accuracy rivals or exceeds that of experienced professionals. But this raises an unsettling question: if the algorithm sees better, should the clinician still look? The result is a quiet bifurcation of roles: clinicians shift from interpreters to verifiers, becoming the *second* reader, not the first. They are still liable for decisions, but increasingly dependent on tools they did not build, cannot audit, and may not fully understand.

The psychological effects of this transition are underexamined but growing. For junior doctors, entering a world where machine predictions precede human assessment alters the developmental arc of expertise. Learning is no longer experiential but comparative: "what did the model say?" becomes the default starting point. For seasoned clinicians, the sense of being second-guessed by an opaque system can corrode confidence and reorient risk aversion. Disagreeing with an algorithm feels less like an exercise of judgment and more like an act of defiance. *Authority becomes not a product of knowledge, but of alignment with the system.*

Resistance to this shift often takes two forms: withdrawal or blind trust. The first is typified by clinicians who avoid AI tools entirely, declining to engage with the outputs they see as intrusive, unaccountable, or misleading. These professionals rely on experience, intuition, and a legacy of practice that feels increasingly out of step with institutional expectations. The second group embraces automation with little scrutiny, accepting AI recommendations as a default and rationalising clinical decisions to match the model. Both paths are dangerous. Withdrawal sidelines valuable data and erodes interdisciplinary relevance. Blind trust risks de-skilling and overfitting to a machine logic that is only as good as its assumptions.

The deeper risk is epistemic: AI does not merely offer answers; it redefines what counts as an answer. A clinician might ask a patient to describe their pain, timing, history, and quality. A predictive model might map that encounter into a probability distribution. These are not competing descriptions—they are incommensurable modes of knowing. The former is situated, relational, and open-ended. The latter is statistical, fixed, and designed to generalise. When decisions must be justified to institutions, insurers, or regulators, the probabilistic frame often wins. *The nuance of clinical narrative is overwritten by the confidence of the numerical.*

This puts clinicians in a bind: either learn to speak the language of the model or risk being sidelined in decisions that are increasingly governed by it. But learning that language—data science, model architecture, output calibration—is not trivial. Most medical curricula do not equip practitioners to critically evaluate AI systems. They are taught anatomy and physiology, not bias propagation or algorithmic drift. As a result, the profession finds itself caught between dependence and disenfranchisement: reliant on systems they did not design, yet unable to meaningfully challenge them.

Consider an oncology department using a predictive model to determine which patients should receive genomic sequencing. The model, trained on historical outcomes, optimises for patients most likely to benefit. On paper, this makes sense—efficient allocation of costly resources. But a seasoned clinician notices a worrying pattern: patients from marginalised backgrounds are underrepresented in the model's selections. Their records are incomplete, their outcomes historically worse, and their cases less likely to match the model's definition of "high benefit." The system does not discriminate maliciously; it simply encodes the biases of past practice. But for the physician who sees this, the options are limited: flag the issue and face pushback, or comply with a tool that systematises inequity. *Expertise, here, becomes a form of ethical risk.*

This tension—between medical judgment and model logic—is compounded by the design of healthcare institutions themselves. Many hospitals now implement algorithmic systems as part of their workflow, billing, or accreditation standards. Once adopted, these tools become difficult to challenge, not because they are flawless, but because they are infrastructural. They are embedded in reporting systems, linked to funding streams, and audited by third parties. The clinician's decision is not merely a medical one—it is embedded in an ecosystem of incentives, liabilities, and algorithmic precedents. *To resist the machine is to resist the institution it supports.*

But it is also true that clinicians are not powerless. There is a window—narrow, but real—for shaping how AI is integrated into practice. Some hospital systems now include clinicians in model validation processes, bias audits, and calibration reviews. Others pair data scientists with physicians to build models that are interpretable, context-sensitive, and sensitive to edge cases. These efforts are early, uneven, and often underfunded. But they represent a counterforce to the trend of obsolescence—a recognition that *clinical knowledge cannot be fully outsourced to code.*

To preserve that knowledge, the medical profession must undergo its own transformation. Not a retreat into tradition, but an expansion into fluency. Clinicians must be able to ask meaningful questions of their tools: What data were you trained on? What assumptions do you carry? What cases fall outside your design scope? Just as a good doctor asks not only *what* but *why*, a good AI-enabled clinician must learn to interrogate the model's reasoning—not to reject it, but to understand its limits.

This kind of fluency does not come from passive exposure. It requires investment in education, cross-disciplinary collaboration, and institutional support for slow thinking in fast systems. It requires reimagining expertise not as a silo of knowledge, but as a capacity to navigate uncertainty—in both human and machine form. And it requires accepting that the future of medical authority will be hybrid: part clinical, part computational, part relational.

The clinician's value is not diminished by AI—it is recontextualised. Expertise will not disappear; it will evolve. The challenge is ensuring that it evolves on terms that preserve its core commitments: to judgment over compliance, to care over efficiency, to accountability over automation. For if expertise becomes synonymous with system conformity, then what is lost is not only professional standing, but the ethical compass that makes medicine a humane art. It is not enough to be accurate. One must still be *right*. And in a world of intelligent systems, *being right requires more than just reading the output—it demands understanding the human stakes behind the prediction.*

Trusting vs. Overruling the Machine

A cardiologist reviews a risk score generated by a predictive algorithm. It suggests that the patient—a 52-year-old woman with a mildly abnormal ECG but no prior cardiac history—has a 7% likelihood of myocardial infarction in the next 30 days. The guideline threshold for hospital admission is 5%. The doctor, however, finds the score inconsistent with her clinical gestalt. The patient is asymptomatic, active, and has no family history. There is nothing in the clinical picture that makes her seem high risk. The algorithm's flag was triggered by a constellation of variables: her age, slight inflammation markers, and a historical correlation pulled from tens of thousands of similar profiles. The physician now faces a silent but pressing choice—*follow the model's recommendation, or trust her clinical judgment?*

This decision—whether to trust or overrule the machine—is becoming one of the defining challenges of modern medicine. Not because artificial intelligence is inherently adversarial to human expertise, but because it recasts the nature of decision-making itself. For centuries, medicine has been practised as a dialogue between experience, evidence, and patient context. AI, by design, introduces a fourth actor: the model. And this actor does not negotiate, explain, or adapt in the human sense. It presents its output—confident, calculated, and data-rich—often without accessible reasoning. The clinician is left to interpret, absorb, or reject, *but rarely to question the internal logic of the machine itself.*

What complicates this further is that these models are frequently right. That is, *statistically* right—better than average in aggregate across thousands of cases. In retrospective studies, AI systems have outperformed humans in areas such as radiological diagnosis, sepsis detection, and stroke triage. And yet, statistical superiority does not translate directly to clinical trust. Real-world decision-making does not operate on averages. It pivots on singularities: *this* patient, *this* presentation, *this* moment. When the algorithm's prediction contradicts the human's intuition, the clinician is not deciding between "science" and "hunch"—they are navigating a contest of epistemologies. *One trained on millions of data points; the other shaped by years of embodied experience and relational care.*

Take, for instance, the case of sepsis alerts in hospital emergency departments. AI-based early warning systems, trained on vast historical data, generate notifications when a patient shows signs that may lead to septic shock. These models have improved mortality rates when implemented well. Yet in practice, clinicians report high alert fatigue—

alarms triggered too frequently, or for patients who don't fit the expected clinical deterioration pattern. Doctors begin to dismiss them, not out of arrogance, but out of calibration. They weigh the cost of action against the credibility of the alert. Trust, here, is not about blind obedience. It is *earned over time, tempered by context, and deeply influenced by workflow design.*

Overruling a machine is not always heroic—it can be a matter of necessity or caution. But it is rarely easy. In many systems, disagreeing with an algorithm requires a formal override process. Justifications must be entered into the electronic health record, often in real time. These workflows create friction—not only cognitive, but administrative. The psychological message is clear: if you wish to go against the system, prepare to explain yourself. *The burden of proof shifts subtly but significantly onto the clinician.* The machine's output becomes the default; human judgment becomes the deviation.

This reversal of clinical hierarchy—where the system's output is treated as the standard rather than a suggestion—has far-reaching consequences. It shapes how doctors think, how they teach, how they document. Medical trainees, in particular, may learn to defer prematurely, treating the algorithm as a primary source rather than a second opinion. The art of critical appraisal is at risk of being replaced by interpretive compliance: understanding *what the model said*, rather than *why it may or may not be reliable.*

This is not an argument against machine learning in medicine. There is no credible future in which computational support is not an integral part of healthcare. But what needs attention is *the quality of interaction* between model and human—the trust dynamic, the space for dialogue, the capacity to disagree intelligently. Effective human-AI collaboration is not a function of accuracy alone. It depends on transparency, calibration, and *design choices that acknowledge the human at the loop, not merely in it.*

Contrast two scenarios. In the first, an oncologist receives a treatment recommendation from an AI trained on genomic data. The recommendation is presented with no accompanying explanation—just a ranked list of therapies. The clinician is left with a binary decision: accept or reject. In the second scenario, the same recommendation includes a visual breakdown of contributing features, comparable cases, confidence intervals, and caveats around data limitations. The second approach doesn't just inform—it educates. It provides the clinician with *a reasoned basis to make a decision, not just a statistical suggestion.*

Explainability, though often difficult to achieve in deep learning models, is not a luxury. It is *a prerequisite for ethical and effective clinical decision-making.* Without it, AI systems may produce correct answers for the wrong reasons—or the right reasons in the wrong context. Clinicians, meanwhile, are left navigating a system that simultaneously demands both trust and accountability, but provides neither clarity nor flexibility in return.

At the heart of this dilemma is a question that remains largely unresolved in current healthcare discourse: *who bears responsibility when the machine is wrong, and the human disagreed but complied?* In most institutional settings, liability still rests with the clinician. But the moral and psychological weight is unevenly distributed. If a physician accepts the machine's recommendation and harm results, the institutional defence may be, "the model was followed." If the physician *rejects* the recommendation and harm results, the defence becomes, "why was the model ignored?" This creates a subtle but pervasive coercion: the safest path is not necessarily the best one—it is the most defensible one.

Over time, such dynamics risk eroding clinical courage. The willingness to act decisively in the face of uncertainty, to stand by a judgment that diverges from consensus or prediction, is not only a mark of expertise—it is a moral commitment. If clinicians lose the latitude to question the system, or are punished for exercising independent reasoning, the profession shifts from one of moral agents to one of procedural operators. *Medicine becomes not an art informed by science, but a protocol governed by probability.*

To resist this flattening of clinical judgement, institutions must design AI systems not as oracles, but as interlocutors. This means building tools that *invite challenge*, offer context, and allow for reversible decisions without penalty. It means training clinicians to ask the right questions of the model, not just to extract the "right" answer. And it means acknowledging that trust is not a static input, but an evolving relationship—a function of experience, outcome, and shared accountability.

There will always be moments when doctors must decide whether to trust the machine or override it. These moments are not failures of design; they are *features* of any system that includes both humans and machines. The challenge is not to eliminate these tensions, but to equip clinicians to navigate them with confidence, competence, and clarity.

The future of medicine depends not just on how well machines predict, but on how well humans *decide*. The clinical voice must remain central—not because it is infallible, but because it is relational, interpretive, and ultimately accountable in ways that machines are not. To trust or to overrule is not a binary choice; it is a clinical act that requires judgment, courage, and an environment that respects both. If we lose sight of this, we risk building systems that are optimised for compliance—but hollowed of care.

Burnout in the Age of Efficiency

Efficiency is often presented as a gift. For overburdened clinicians navigating time-starved hospital corridors and labyrinthine documentation systems, the promise of automation reads like a balm: fewer clicks, faster triage, smarter diagnostics, reduced error. Artificial intelligence enters this equation with a compelling narrative—it will relieve physicians of the menial and administrative so they can focus on the human. But reality, as it plays out in clinics, emergency rooms, and consultation lounges, tells a more sobering story. Far from alleviating cognitive and bureaucratic strain, many AI-integrated systems are compounding it. *The very tools designed to unburden are subtly reshaping the work of medicine into a form that is more fragmented, more surveilled, and more exhausting.*

At first glance, this seems counterintuitive. Why should more data, better automation, and predictive algorithms increase burnout rather than reduce it? The answer lies in how these systems are designed, implemented, and justified—not as support mechanisms, but as productivity engines. The underlying ethos is not care but throughput. AI, in most institutional settings, is not framed as a colleague but as a metric-generating machine, amplifying the already dehumanising pressures of performance targets and billing frameworks. The clinician is not so much augmented as audited.

A 2023 cross-sectional study published in *JAMA Internal Medicine* found that the use of AI-assisted diagnostic tools in primary care was associated with increased documentation time per patient, rather than a reduction. The software automatically generated suggested text and clinical justifications, but clinicians were still responsible for reviewing, editing, and validating every line. The result: more time on screens, less time with patients, and growing resentment toward a system that had promised the opposite. *Efficiency in theory became labour in practice.*

This disconnect between intention and experience is magnified by the creeping expansion of cognitive overhead. AI systems often require clinicians to learn new interfaces, interpret complex outputs, and engage in layers of data validation that did not previously exist. A radiologist, once trained to interpret scans visually and narratively, may now need to evaluate risk scores, cross-reference model weights, and troubleshoot integration errors. The time spent understanding what the model is doing—and whether it is doing it correctly—is rarely offset by equivalent reductions in core workload. Instead, *the machine adds a parallel task-stream that mimics assistance but feels more like delegation without relief.*

Even more insidious is the psychological load introduced by what might be called *ambient accountability*. AI-infused systems capture not just clinical decisions but meta-decisions: how long a physician reviews a file, which recommendations they accept or reject, how quickly they respond to alerts. These behaviours are logged, monitored, and sometimes scored. The clinician begins to feel like a data subject within the very systems meant to support them. Every keystroke becomes a potential audit trail. This is not empowerment; it is a digital form of managerialism that corrodes professional autonomy while claiming to optimise it.

There is also the matter of emotional labour, often overlooked in discussions of clinical burnout. AI does not absorb this load; it often multiplies it. Consider the use of chatbots in triage systems. Patients interact with a conversational interface that collects symptoms and generates preliminary assessments before the clinician even enters the room. On paper, this improves efficiency. In reality, it introduces subtle but profound disruptions to the therapeutic encounter. The physician must reconcile the bot's structured intake with the patient's own narrative, which may contradict or complicate the machine's version. This negotiation is not trivial. It requires time, tact, and often, re-explanation. *Clinicians are not just treating illness—they are translating systems back into human terms.*

The broader irony is that these technologies are being deployed in an environment already structurally misaligned with human flourishing. Burnout in medicine is not new. It predates AI and is driven by multiple forces: understaffing, moral distress, misaligned incentives, relentless documentation, and the commodification of care. But AI doesn't arrive into a neutral space—it lands in the middle of a crisis and risks being weaponised by the very structures that caused it. When tools designed to relieve become tools to extract, *what we call innovation becomes a form of intensification.*

Some might argue that this is a transitional problem—that as systems mature, interfaces improve, and workflows stabilise, the burdens will recede. But this assumes that the problem lies in technology alone. It does not. The deeper issue is institutional culture: the demand that clinicians become more productive without becoming more supported. AI fits too neatly into this mandate. It offers the illusion of capacity without the investment in care. It promises performance without addressing the human cost. *What we face is not a failure of machine learning—it is a failure of organisational imagination.*

There are counterexamples worth examining. In some integrated health systems, AI has been deployed in explicitly restorative ways. At the Mayo Clinic, predictive models have been used to preemptively flag patients at risk of hospital readmission—not to penalise clinicians, but to mobilise social workers, follow-up care, and community resources. These systems work because they are embedded in a culture that values support over surveillance. Similarly, in some Scandinavian health systems, clinicians have been involved in the co-design of AI tools, ensuring that outputs align with actual workflows rather than abstract productivity metrics. *These are not technological solutions; they are relational strategies enabled by technology.*

If AI is to serve as a balm rather than a burden, it must be developed with a different kind of efficiency in mind—not one measured in clicks saved or tasks automated, but in *relational integrity preserved*. This means protecting time for reflection, ensuring the interpretability of outputs, and giving clinicians the authority to shape how tools are used. It also means recognising that not all inefficiencies are problems to be solved. Some are forms of care. The long pause in a consultation, the seemingly redundant note in a patient record, the informal conversation between shifts—these are not artefacts to be optimised away. They are the texture of human work.

The current trajectory risks hollowing this texture in favour of technical elegance. AI is not neutral in how it reshapes time, attention, or moral labour. And while the technologies themselves may be evolving, the systems into which they are embedded are often ossified by design. To pretend that digital tools alone will fix burnout is to mistake a structural wound for a user interface glitch.

What's required, then, is not merely better tools, but *better questions*: Who benefits from this efficiency? Who defines the metrics? Who absorbs the cognitive fallout of failed automation? And most importantly, who gets to decide what counts as meaningful work in medicine?

Until those questions are addressed with clarity, courage, and compassion, AI will remain what it increasingly feels like to many clinicians—not a support, but a shadow: always present, always watching, and always asking for more. The path forward lies not in resisting technology, but in resisting the logic that treats clinicians as inputs to be optimised rather than professionals to be empowered. Only then can the promise of artificial intelligence begin to feel like *relief*, rather than another name for relentless demand.

Training the Machine, Losing the Craft

A generation ago, a seasoned physician could often identify a brewing illness before a diagnostic test ever confirmed it. Not through clairvoyance, but through the slow accumulation of clinical intuition—a craft honed over thousands of patient interactions, embedded in memory, gesture, language, and silence. This tacit knowledge, the ability to detect what isn't immediately visible, remains the lifeblood of medicine. Yet increasingly, that craft is being displaced—outsourced to algorithms, nudged aside by probabilistic models, and redefined by a data-centric logic that favours measurable signals over embodied sense. *As clinicians become trainers of machines, they risk becoming untrained in themselves.*

Artificial intelligence in medicine is not inherently antithetical to human skill. But the way it is often implemented reorients the structure of medical thinking. Tasks that once required clinical judgement are now mediated by pattern recognition tools that present results as "smart" defaults. A chest scan flagged by a deep learning model as showing "moderate probability of embolism" exerts a subtle coercion. It does not demand obedience outright, but it recasts human evaluation as a potential deviation from statistical reasoning. In this dynamic, the clinician becomes the outlier, not the algorithm. *The very tools built to support expertise risk undermining its authority.*

This recalibration of decision-making carries epistemic consequences. When AI systems become arbiters of diagnosis and risk, they create a new normativity—what they see becomes what matters. Training datasets, built on historical records, encode past clinical decisions and population averages. But these are not neutral references; they are shaped by systemic biases, documentation habits, and institutional blind spots. Clinicians, working alongside these tools, are asked not only to use the machine but to help refine it—label data, correct outputs, validate predictions. Over time, their role tilts toward that of supervisor and annotator, rather than autonomous practitioner. *They teach the system, but unlearn the felt complexity of real-life care.*

This shift is most visible in domains where the affective dimension of medicine has traditionally played a central role. In psychiatry, for example, natural language processing tools are being developed to extract "depression indicators" from speech patterns, or predict suicidality from social media posts. These technologies are impressive in scope, but brittle in texture. They do not listen the way a psychiatrist listens: for hesitations, self-contradictions, layered meaning, and cultural nuance. They hear language as data, not dialogue. As such tools proliferate, clinicians are being encouraged to interpret affect as metadata—a trend that narrows their interpretive gaze. *The risk is not just diagnostic error; it is empathic erosion.*

The erosion is rarely explicit. It shows up in small shifts: in the structuring of clinical interviews around data capture, in the shortening of narrative space during consultations, in the quiet pressure to defer to model output when time is tight. Over time, these shifts produce a form of epistemic dependency. Clinicians begin to trust their own judgement less—not because they lack skill, but because the system no longer rewards or reinforces it. In hospital settings where decisions must be documented and defensible, defying an algorithm requires not just confidence, but administrative courage. *The path of least resistance is paved with compliance.*

Meanwhile, the feedback loop tightens. As more clinicians rely on model-assisted decisions, the data generated from these choices feeds the next generation of models. But this feedback is filtered through the same structural lens. False positives, ambiguous cases, and subtle diagnoses that once expanded a physician's heuristic repertoire are now less likely to be recorded in meaningful ways. Instead, the system codifies what is confirmable, binary, and legible to the machine. The full arc of clinical discernment is compressed into a labelled output. *In training the machine to approximate human reasoning, we gradually narrow the boundaries of what that reasoning is allowed to be.*

This is not merely a technical concern—it is a philosophical one. What does it mean to practise medicine when your primary decisions are being continuously framed, corrected, or overruled by a non-human intelligence? What happens to moral responsibility when actions are co-authored by systems whose logic cannot be fully interrogated? The clinician's role shifts from moral agent to procedural intermediary. They become the one who clicks 'approve', not the one who listens, deliberates, and decides. *And yet, when outcomes go wrong, accountability remains resolutely human.*

There are countercurrents that push back against this tide. Some teaching hospitals are developing curricula that explicitly address AI fluency—not simply as technical literacy, but as a lens for critical thinking. These programmes aim to help future doctors understand what models can do, but also what they obscure. Others advocate for *inverse training*, where clinicians periodically practise diagnosis without digital augmentation, much like pilots rehearse manual flight. These exercises are not nostalgic rituals—they are recalibrations of agency. *They remind practitioners that clinical intuition is not a relic but a renewable form of intelligence.*

Still, these are exceptions, not norms. The dominant trend across many healthcare systems is towards hyper-documentation, hyper-codification, and a procedural logic that treats ambiguity as inefficiency. In such a context, relational care becomes harder to sustain. It is not that clinicians forget how to connect with patients—it is that the system de-incentivises the time and reflection required to do so. And when intuition is no longer part of the workflow, it begins to atrophy.

Consider the experience of a senior nurse practitioner in a London hospital who described feeling increasingly alienated from younger colleagues trained under AI-integrated systems. "They're brilliant at navigating protocols," she said, "but less confident with uncertainty. They don't probe as much. If the system says it's fine, they move on." This is not a deficit of intelligence—it is a consequence of environmental conditioning. When exploration is not modelled or rewarded, it recedes. *We do not lose the craft all at once. We forget that it is missing.*

Ultimately, the question is not whether machines should assist clinicians. Of course they should. The question is whether we are building systems that assist without replacing, that support without eroding. Clinical wisdom is not reducible to best practices or decision trees. It is situational, lived, and intuitive. It emerges from contradiction, from what is not written down. And it cannot be fully transferred to a model whose logic depends on past patterns and predefined labels.

To preserve this wisdom, institutions must revalue the intangible: the moment of doubt, the instinct to ask again, the pause that precedes the unexpected question. These are not inefficiencies—they are the muscle fibres of good medicine. If AI is to be a partner in care, it must learn to respect them. More importantly, *we must remember to protect them.*

Because once we forget how to listen without a model, to notice without a prompt, to care without a prompt—what we lose is not just a method. We lose medicine itself.

Chapter 7
Designing for Dignity

Technology, in truth, is never neutral. The configuration of a hospital ward, the pacing of a digital interface, the drop-down choices in an electronic health record—these are not incidental; they are deliberate design decisions that shape experience, exert influence, and embed values. In healthcare, where outcomes are inseparable from the manner in which care is delivered, these choices carry ethical significance. Designing an AI system is never merely technical—it is moral. Whether a patient feels acknowledged or handled, respected or reduced, often hinges less on the precision of the algorithm than on the environment it cultivates for human interaction.

Designing for dignity is not decoration or sentiment; it is a conscious refusal to accept dehumanisation as the price of efficiency. It treats interface choices as moral expressions, not just workflow optimisations. A predictive tool labelling a patient "noncompliant" without context may streamline operations, but it flattens a life into a metric. A triage system that ranks by statistical risk without room for narrative may move patients quickly, but it does not attend to them. Design either magnifies dignity or diminishes it—there is no middle ground.

Much of contemporary healthcare AI remains model-centred. Systems optimise for performance metrics that rarely capture what matters most to patients: being understood, retaining agency, preserving privacy, receiving care attuned to emotional and cultural nuances. These concerns are often dismissed as "soft" or "non-clinical," conveniently placed beyond the scope of evaluation. But this is a fundamental misstep: respect is not a luxury; it is the foundation of trust.

Friction emerges because AI and clinical practice often operate on different epistemologies. Medicine constructs meaning at the point of contact—doctor and patient, story and symptom. Data informs but does not replace this interaction. Yet most AI tools are developed with minimal engagement from those they aim to serve. Consequently, many systems operate *on* patients rather than *with* them, optimising prediction over participation.

Co-creation offers an alternative. When patients, clinicians, and designers collaborate from the outset, the result is not only more humane technology, but more effective technology. Take a Scandinavian cancer centre where young adults worked directly with technologists to design an AI support system. Standard symptom checklists were rejected in favour of narrative prompts; conversational, rather than clinical, language was insisted upon; emotional distress was routed to trained peer counsellors rather than emergency services. The system monitored health, yes, but it honoured context.

Yet such examples are exceptional. More often, AI systems are deployed with little adaptation to ethical, cultural, or interpersonal realities. Success is measured by aggregate metrics: reduced readmissions, improved throughput, compliance with protocol. These figures can obscure as much as they reveal. A drop in face-to-face consultations may appear efficient, but at what human cost? Without mechanisms to capture meaning, crucial trade-offs remain unseen. What gets measured may be managed; what truly matters can slip through the cracks.

Metrics themselves are not the enemy—but they must be complemented by qualitative insight. Error rates and satisfaction scores tell only part of the story. They cannot capture the moral texture of care: the tone of an encounter, whether a patient felt heard, whether cultural knowledge was respected. Forward-looking health systems experiment with composite measures, blending clinical data with narrative feedback, peer evaluation, and community input. Imperfect, perhaps, but principled. The aim is not objectivity alone, but integrity married to meaning.

Patient autonomy is another casualty of careless design. Many AI tools subtly shift decision-making away from the individual under the guise of assistance. A diabetes app nudging specific behaviours may enhance control, yet restrict flexibility. A mental health chatbot may increase access, yet supplant human dialogue and silence nuance. Technology that denies the right to question, resist, or reinterpret is not empowering—it is paternalistic.

True patient-centred design asks not only what patients need, but how they wish to be cared for. It requires an ethics of invitation: openness to redesign, renegotiation, and responsiveness. Humility is essential—acknowledging that expertise is distributed, not centralised. Patients inhabit the systems we build; they notice where pain accumulates, dignity leaks, and design fails. Ignoring their insights is not inefficiency—it is injustice.

Designing for dignity also requires embracing pluralism. Respect in one context may feel intrusive in another. Cultural values, language, historical trauma—all shape experience. Facial recognition in an emergency ward may streamline check-ins for some, yet evoke surveillance and mistrust for others. A genetic risk predictor may trigger proactive screening while imposing psychological and social burdens. Ethical design must anticipate such tensions; uniform solutions in diverse societies are not neutral—they exclude.

The future of healthcare AI will be defined not merely by what we can build, but by what we choose to build. Predicting hospitalisations or optimising adherence is possible; the question is whether we can do so while upholding dignity, preserving narrative space, honouring diversity, and strengthening relational care. This is a design challenge, an ethical imperative, a political choice.

No interface is neutral enough to absolve us of responsibility. Every button, prompt, dashboard carries ideology. Every workflow empowers or constrains. Language, defaults, feedback—these are not afterthoughts; they are moral acts. In healthcare, design is never just about usability. It shapes who gets to feel human in the act of being treated.

This chapter engages with these questions seriously. It examines what it means to design *with* patients, not merely for them. It interrogates the boundary between optimisation and empathy. It considers how systems might measure not just efficiency, but meaning. At its core, this is not a technical conversation—it is a moral one. Patient dignity is not an emergent property of software; it must be deliberately built from the start.

Ethics by Design

The ethical character of a system is not defined by its intentions but by its architecture. In healthcare, where decisions affect vulnerability, mortality, and meaning, design is not merely functional—it is moral infrastructure. Artificial intelligence introduces unprecedented speed, complexity, and reach to this space, yet its ethical foundations often remain an afterthought. The assumption persists that ethical review can be appended to finished systems, as though autonomy, empathy, and cultural nuance are UX filters rather than structural commitments. *This is not a failure of imagination; it is a failure of responsibility.*

Most AI systems in healthcare are built to optimise measurable outcomes: risk prediction, diagnostic accuracy, resource allocation. These goals are not inherently unethical, but *what they exclude often is.* A triage tool that assigns lower urgency to patients with limited English proficiency because they report symptoms less fluently may deliver efficient throughput—while systematically disadvantaging a linguistic minority. A hospital chatbot that offers appointment reminders but ignores the emotional tone of patient messages may seem "scalable"—yet leave psychological distress unacknowledged. *Designs that streamline process while silencing personhood are not ethical oversights; they are engineered erasures.*

Respecting autonomy in AI design does not mean merely offering choices. It means creating systems that honour the *conditions* for choice: clarity, deliberation, informed context, and the right to dissent. Consider a wearable that prompts hypertensive patients to take their medication based on biometric data. Without context about the user's environment—work demands, side effects, food availability—the nudge becomes coercion masked as care. Worse, if the interface is designed to discourage override, or if deviation triggers alerts to third parties, autonomy is actively subverted. *Ethics by design begins with the presumption that human agency must not be automated away for convenience.*

Empathy is often treated as non-essential in digital health tools—a trait desirable in physicians, dispensable in software. This is a profound misreading of how people process care. Clinical effectiveness does not happen in a vacuum; it is relationally mediated. Interfaces that ignore tone, context, or affect can easily deliver correct information in ways that produce alienation. For instance, a cancer risk calculator that bluntly states, "Your 5-year probability of recurrence is 67%" may be mathematically sound—but if delivered via a sterile screen without interpretive support, it functions more as existential violence than as empowerment. *An ethically designed system communicates in ways calibrated not only to accuracy, but to emotional salience and psychological safety.*

Cultural nuance in AI design is not a matter of localisation or aesthetic inclusion—it is about embedding systems with the *cultural literacy* necessary to interpret human variation meaningfully. For example, pain expression differs substantially across cultures; so do attitudes toward authority, disclosure, and uncertainty. An AI trained on datasets from Western clinical encounters may interpret stoicism as absence of symptoms or deference as diagnostic ambiguity. Similarly, risk calculators that use ethnicity as a proxy variable often bake in historical discrimination without critical interrogation. *Cultural sensitivity is not a plug-in; it is a fundamental design question: whose reality is normalised, whose is flagged, and whose is ignored?*

Too often, ethical design is conflated with regulatory compliance. But the ability to pass legal muster is not the same as moral adequacy. Data protection laws may require user consent for tracking, but they do not ask whether the act of surveillance itself is experienced as invasive. An app may be HIPAA-compliant yet still generate anxiety through opaque scoring, gamified health metrics, or reductive summaries. True ethical design *does not wait for permission; it anticipates discomfort, resists simplification, and builds with care as a constraint.*

Real-world case studies demonstrate how intentional ethical design can reshape patient experiences. A telepsychiatry startup in New Zealand, for example, restructured its onboarding process after community consultation with Māori patients. Rather than standardised intake forms, they designed conversational pathways that began with ancestral and familial questions—restoring the cultural rhythm of introduction known as *whakawhanaungatanga*. The result was not only higher engagement, but deeper clinical rapport. *The ethics were not in the content—they were in the interface, the sequencing, the logic of respect.*

Contrast this with mainstream symptom checkers that assume universality. Many present users with drop-down menus for gender: "male," "female," "prefer not to say." A nonbinary user confronted with this menu has already been excluded before data entry begins. More subtly, tools that track menstrual cycles or fertility assume cisgender usage patterns, reinforcing biological essentialism. These may seem like edge cases to designers focused on scale—but *designs that ignore the margins inevitably reinforce majoritarian norms*.

Ethical design also involves resisting overreach. Just because AI can be integrated into a clinical task does not mean it should. In palliative care, for instance, the appeal of predictive models for forecasting end-of-life trajectories is clear. But how does one design an interface that delivers news of impending mortality without fracturing the patient's sense of control, hope, or humanity? No algorithm can ethically convey such news without a human interpretive frame. *Design ethics means knowing when the machine must defer to the moment's emotional gravity.*

Transparency is frequently proposed as a universal remedy—make algorithms interpretable, and trust will follow. But *transparency is not trustworthiness*. A radiology AI may expose its saliency map or confidence interval, but if it cannot explain *why* it recommended against a biopsy in language that resonates with the clinician's experience and the patient's concern, transparency serves little ethical function. The question is not just whether a system can be explained, but *to whom*, *in what context*, and *with what consequence*. Ethical design prioritises communicability—not just code legibility, but conversational clarity.

There are practical design principles that reflect these commitments, though none offer shortcuts. Ethical AI design in healthcare must begin with multi-stakeholder input: *not just* domain experts and technologists, but patients, caregivers, social workers, and ethicists. Participatory design processes—where users are not only testers but co-architects—yield systems that reflect lived experience, not just statistical abstraction. Iteration must include feedback on emotional resonance, language usability, and potential for harm. Usability testing should be paired with *vulnerability audits*: how might this system disempower, misrepresent, or retraumatise?

Accountability must also be embedded at the design layer. Systems should include friction by design—moments where users must pause, review, and reflect. A clinical decision-support tool, for example, might flag uncertainty rather than enforce protocol: "The recommendation is based on limited data for patients over 75—consider reviewing with caution." This is not inefficiency; it is *ethically productive hesitation*. Similarly, designers can build in opt-out pathways that are not buried in complexity. A user's right to disengage is a litmus test for ethical integrity.

There are no perfect designs, only *intentional* ones. Trade-offs are inevitable. Every design encodes values—efficiency over deliberation, standardisation over nuance, automation over discretion. Ethical design makes these trade-offs visible, discussable, and contestable. It invites revision rather than foreclosing it. It treats harm as a possibility to be mitigated, not a risk to be actuarially accepted. And it orients systems toward people as *subjects of care*, not objects of optimisation.

In healthcare, dignity is not a secondary consideration. It is the atmosphere in which everything else—diagnosis, treatment, recovery—takes place. Systems that erode dignity erode trust, engagement, and adherence. No level of precision can compensate for alienation. *To design ethically is to design relationally.* It is to ask, at every turn, not only *"Is this efficient?"* or *"Is this accurate?"* but *"Is this respectful?" "Is this equitable?" "Is this humanising?"*

These are not abstract questions. They are the questions that shape how people experience the most intimate, vulnerable, and consequential moments of their lives. That is what is at stake in ethics by design. Not compliance. Not usability. *Care.*

Patient-Centered vs. Model-Centered Care

The promise of artificial intelligence in healthcare is seductive: faster diagnoses, fewer errors, more efficient workflows. But beneath the surface of that technological optimism lies a structural tension that is redefining what it means to care. At the heart of the modern clinical encounter, a quiet battle is unfolding between two paradigms—one that centres the patient as a complex human being, and another that centres the model as an optimiser of probabilities. These paradigms are not always in conflict, but when they are, the interface becomes the battleground, and the stakes are not simply operational—they are moral.

Interfaces shape behaviour. They mediate attention, establish hierarchies, and structure what gets seen, said, and acted upon. In clinical environments, they have the power to elevate a patient's narrative—or render it invisible. When electronic health records (EHRs), decision-support tools, and predictive dashboards are designed primarily around model logic—standardised fields, algorithmic flags, alert hierarchies—there is little space left for the patient's voice. Notes become checkboxes. Symptoms become dropdowns. Uncertainty becomes a red flag. *The clinician's screen becomes a cognitive tunnel, narrowing focus to what the model prioritises, rather than what the patient expresses.*

Consider the experience of a general practitioner seeing a patient with chronic fatigue. The patient describes fluctuating symptoms, emotional stressors, and a sense of being dismissed by past providers. The GP opens the EHR and is immediately met with a best-practice alert suggesting screening for depression, based on prior notes and current keywords. A predictive module proposes a workup for anaemia, citing population-level correlations. What the interface doesn't capture—or incentivise—is the narrative nuance: that the patient's experience is shaped by caregiving responsibilities, cultural stigma, and the accumulation of medical mistrust. The interface is model-centred; it directs the clinician toward algorithmically ranked pathways while relegating human context to an optional sidebar. *In doing so, it subtly redefines what counts as legitimate input—and what becomes digital noise.*

This tension is not new. Medicine has long oscillated between reductionism and holism, between treating data and treating persons. But what makes the current moment distinctive is the sheer scale and speed at which model logic can overtake clinical judgment. AI-powered systems are not neutral tools—they are infrastructures that organise clinical cognition. A triage interface that prioritises patients based on vital sign thresholds may exclude those whose symptoms are serious but don't trigger model alerts. A risk score that flags noncompliance based on pharmacy refills may penalise patients who skip medication for economic or cultural reasons. These systems are not just influencing care—they are *reframing the definition of need.*

Design decisions become ethical decisions. When the patient's subjective voice is decoupled from the system's operational logic, it becomes harder for clinicians to advocate effectively. Many interface workflows make it burdensome to document complexity, override recommendations, or explore non-algorithmic paths. In busy clinical environments, friction leads to conformity. And conformity, in turn, rewards the model—not the patient. *Over time, the very texture of clinical care risks being reshaped to accommodate the system, rather than the story.*

Yet patient-centred design is not simply a matter of adding open text boxes or digital empathy prompts. It requires a deeper structural reorientation—one that treats the patient not merely as a data source, but as a co-interpreter of meaning. In a model-centred world, the system seeks patterns in populations; in a patient-centred one, the goal is understanding in context. This means designing workflows that make space for narrative, ambiguity, and deliberation. It means building interfaces that allow disagreement—not just between clinicians and systems, but between patients and recommendations. *Ethical care requires interpretive space, not just predictive accuracy.*

There are instructive examples. In some community health settings, patient-owned records have been designed to foreground personal goals and values—not just clinical metrics. Instead of a dashboard displaying blood glucose and BMI trends alone, the interface begins with the patient's own priorities: "I want to walk my daughter to school without pain." The clinical data is contextualised within that aspiration, not outside of it. Care plans are co-authored. This shifts the orientation from compliance to collaboration, from adherence to meaning. *Design becomes a means of preserving agency, not enforcing conformity.*

Contrast this with hospital systems where patient voices are translated into algorithmic input but never returned in human-readable form. A patient may answer dozens of intake questions, submit biometric data, and complete validated mental health scales—only to receive a canned message or a generic care path. They are visible to the model but invisible to the clinician. Their data flows, but their story stalls. *In such systems, personalisation is operational but not relational. It is tailored care without felt understanding.*

The issue is not that models are incapable of supporting human care. On the contrary, they can be powerful allies—when subordinated to clinical discretion and patient voice. But when models become proxies for care itself—when they set the agenda, define the thresholds, and suggest the only relevant options—they risk reconstituting patients as *problems to be solved*, not *persons to be heard*. This is not a trivial shift. It changes how illness is framed, how responsibility is assigned, and how healing is imagined.

It is also important to recognise the seductive logic of scale. Model-centred systems are scalable; they promise uniformity, replicability, and cost-efficiency. Patient-centred care, by contrast, is often local, relational, and time-intensive. It requires listening, interpreting, and adapting. The temptation, then, is to treat patient-centredness as a luxury—an ideal for the privileged few or the exceptional cases. But *ethical systems are not built on averages*. They are judged by how well they accommodate difference, dissent, and unpredictability. The very patients who fall through the cracks of model logic are often those who most need personalised attention.

There is a broader philosophical question here: What is the epistemic authority of the patient in AI-mediated care? Are they informants, collaborators, or end-users? If design treats patients as inputs into optimisation functions, their voice is conditional—validated only insofar as it confirms the model's assumptions. If, instead, design begins from the presumption that *subjective experience is indispensable*, then every interface, every alert, every prompt must be scrutinised for how it either amplifies or mutes that experience.

Clinicians, too, must be supported to act as interpreters, not just operators. Interfaces that foreground model recommendations without equally foregrounding patient context risk narrowing clinical attention. A predictive suggestion to initiate anticoagulation may be statistically sound, but if the patient has cultural reservations, logistical barriers, or prior trauma, the human cost of adherence may far exceed the clinical benefit. *Designing for concordance, not just compliance, demands tools that visualise trade-offs, not just outputs.*

It is possible to imagine—and build—systems that make patient-centred care the default, not the exception. Interfaces can be designed to surface questions, not just answers. Dashboards can prioritise *what matters to the patient*, not merely what is measurable. AI recommendations can be nested within interpretive scaffolds that invite reflection, not automation. When patients see their voice reflected in the system—not just in token gestures, but in functional logic—they are more likely to trust, engage, and collaborate. *The system becomes not just technically intelligent, but relationally competent.*

Ultimately, patient-centred care is not a design aesthetic. It is a moral stance. It insists that care is not reducible to metrics, pathways, or probabilities. It reminds us that medicine, at its best, is a practice of attunement—a shared effort to make sense of suffering, restore dignity, and navigate uncertainty. Interfaces and workflows are not peripheral to that work—they are the grammar in which it is written. Whether that grammar speaks in the language of models or in the cadence of human stories will shape the future of care itself.

Co-Creation in System Design

The notion that healthcare technologies should be co-designed with those they affect is often voiced but rarely realised. In practice, system design tends to favour efficiency, technical feasibility, and institutional convenience over lived experience. The resulting platforms—be they patient portals, electronic health records, or AI-driven triage tools—reflect the logics of those who build them rather than those who must use them. Yet, when patients, clinicians, and technologists come together not as stakeholders to be "consulted" but as equals in the design process, a different kind of system emerges: one grounded in empathy, relevance, and moral imagination.

This shift is not merely about better user interfaces or more inclusive surveys. It is a philosophical reorientation that asks: *Whose expertise matters? Whose voice shapes the system?* Traditional design methodologies privilege computational logic and institutional norms. Co-creation invites a different set of questions: What does it feel like to be a patient navigating uncertainty? What cognitive burdens do clinicians face when switching between a screen and a suffering person? What hidden assumptions are embedded in a model's definitions of success?

A case worth examining is the development of MyPath, a collaborative decision-support tool piloted in an oncology setting in Canada. Rather than beginning with the software architecture or predictive modelling, the project started with conversations—deep, facilitated dialogues between patients undergoing chemotherapy, their caregivers, oncologists, nurses, and digital developers. Patients spoke not only of treatment regimens but of fatigue that undermined parenting, of pain that wasn't recorded in standardised scales, and of anxiety triggered by ambiguous clinical notes. Technologists listened. Clinicians challenged their own assumptions. What emerged was not a system optimised for throughput but a tool designed to help patients articulate values and goals, then visualise how treatment options aligned—or failed to align—with them.

Unlike many decision aids, MyPath did not present the "best" option. It presented *trade-offs*, contextualised by the patient's own words. The system's interface was built around narrative snippets, not just data points. When patients saw their language reflected back, when clinicians saw summaries embedded with direct quotations and ethical tensions, dialogue improved. Treatment decisions became more collaborative. *The system was not a replacement for clinical judgment or patient choice—it was a facilitator of mutual understanding.*

Contrast this with typical AI systems deployed in hospital emergency departments. Risk scores are calculated, stratified, and flagged for action—without the patient ever knowing. Clinicians are expected to trust or contest these scores under time pressure. Patients are reduced to input vectors; their preferences, histories, and anxieties are rarely part of the computational equation. Even when designers conduct "user testing," it often focuses on whether clinicians can *use* the tool, not whether they feel it aligns with the ethical core of their practice.

The difference with co-creation is the *relational architecture.* In a project at the University of Washington, a team designing a symptom tracker for long COVID patients refused to assume what "recovery" meant. Instead, they built ethnographic interviews and peer-led workshops into the design process. Patients didn't just describe symptoms—they contested definitions. What clinicians interpreted as anxiety was, in some cases, the patient's acute awareness of physiological changes not yet recognised by diagnostic tools. Rather than correcting patient narratives with medical labels, the system allowed dual entries: clinician interpretation alongside patient framing. *This choice—minor in code but major in philosophy—reflected a commitment to epistemic humility.*

Such humility is difficult to encode in systems driven by optimisation metrics. That is why co-creation must begin before code is written. The dominant model in healthcare innovation remains top-down: researchers develop an intervention, test it on users, and refine based on feedback. Co-creation disrupts that logic. It recognises that patients and front-line clinicians are not just recipients of technology—they are *experts in constraint, friction, and meaning*. Their insights are not "qualitative noise" but *design imperatives.*

In the Dutch initiative "ZorgSamen" (CareTogether), primary care providers and patients with multimorbidity co-developed a planning tool to replace fragmented care plans issued by various specialists. Rather than merely integrating data from multiple sources, the project sought to integrate values. Patients expressed frustration with contradictory advice—exercise from one specialist conflicted with bedrest from another; a diet plan ignored food insecurity; medication changes overlapped dangerously. By mapping these realities with patients and clinicians in joint workshops, the design team created a coordination platform that did not seek to resolve contradictions algorithmically. Instead, it made them visible—so that care discussions could start from the lived complexity, not an artificial clarity imposed by the system.

The result? Not flawless care, but more *honest* care. Patients felt seen. Clinicians felt less pressured to defend protocols that didn't fit. And most importantly, the system gained legitimacy not through mandates, but through shared authorship. *Technology becomes humane not through sleek design, but through deep collaboration.*

Critically, co-creation is not the same as user acceptance testing or focus groups. It demands a redistribution of authority. In a Stanford Health AI project attempting to integrate natural language processing into mental health triage, the team faced early pushback from therapists who felt the tool undermined their relational skills. Rather than shelving the project or overriding dissent, the design team invited therapists to co-write model guardrails. They collaboratively defined when and how AI should intervene—and when it should remain silent. The end product was not just more accurate; it was *more respectful of the therapeutic frame.*

Such efforts are time-intensive. They are not always scalable in the conventional sense. But they offer something rarely found in standard innovation cycles: *moral legitimacy*. When patients are asked not just "what do you think of this tool?" but "what should this tool *do*, and *why*?" the answers often challenge foundational assumptions. In a paediatrics project in rural India, mothers rejected a symptom checker's ranking logic because it prioritised fever severity over feeding ability—an indicator they viewed as more culturally and contextually meaningful. The development team pivoted. They reweighted metrics based on maternal input. The final tool was not just more locally relevant—it achieved higher usage and greater trust, precisely because it *honoured local knowledge*.

What co-creation demands, ultimately, is a recalibration of what counts as expertise. It insists that technologists learn from narrative, not just numbers; that clinicians accept patients as co-navigators of uncertainty; and that patients see themselves not as subjects of care, but *partners in design*. This is not sentiment—it is strategy. Systems designed with users tend to work better *because they reflect the complexity of actual life*, not idealised models.

Of course, co-creation is not a panacea. It can be performative. It can be co-opted. Tokenistic participation risks reinforcing power asymmetries rather than dismantling them. That is why *structure matters*: clear mechanisms for shared decision-making, transparent processes for design trade-offs, and reflexive practices for interrogating whose voices dominate. True co-creation is uncomfortable. It slows things down. But it also deepens trust and surfaces needs that no market analysis or machine learning pipeline will detect.

In an era where healthcare systems are under pressure to do more with less, there is a risk that co-creation will be deemed too costly, too inefficient. But that judgement rests on a narrow view of value. *A system that fails to account for patients' lived realities is efficient only in theory.* Co-creation offers an alternative route—not slower innovation, but wiser innovation. Systems built with humility and solidarity may not be flawless, but they will be more just.

That is the design challenge we face: not just to build tools that work, but to build systems that care—*and know how to care well*. Co-creation is not a luxury. It is a discipline of attention, a stance of respect, and a method of making meaning together. If humane technology is our goal, shared authorship must be our means.

Beyond Metrics: Measuring Meaningful Outcomes

A patient walks into a hospital and receives a timely diagnosis, an evidence-based treatment, and a discharge within the benchmarked 72-hour window. Every box on the quality assurance checklist is ticked. On paper, the system has worked. But the patient leaves with questions unanswered, symptoms unexplained, and a gnawing sense of invisibility. The metrics are satisfied; the experience is not. This dissonance reveals a growing fault line in modern healthcare: *when efficiency becomes a proxy for care, the immeasurable dimensions of healing begin to disappear.*

The dominance of quantifiable indicators in healthcare is neither accidental nor entirely misguided. In overburdened systems, measurable outcomes—readmission rates, time-to-treatment, infection rates—offer a semblance of accountability. They allow regulators to compare hospitals, insurers to allocate resources, and administrators to optimise workflows. But beneath this logic lies an epistemic narrowing. *What can be measured is prioritised; what cannot be measured is sidelined.* And increasingly, the tools that define healthcare performance—especially AI-driven analytics—further entrench this bias.

Consider how predictive algorithms are trained: they rely on structured, historical data. This means that whatever is routinely documented—lab values, imaging results, ICD codes—shapes what counts as a meaningful signal. Yet much of what matters to patients is not documented at all: how safe they felt, whether they understood their diagnosis, whether the care aligned with their personal values. These dimensions resist standardisation, not because they are unimportant, but because they are *qualitative, contingent, and embodied.*

Take the example of palliative care. A patient with late-stage cancer may technically "fail" certain metrics—pain scores may not reach zero, length of stay may exceed targets—but the goal is not cure; it is *dignity*. Measuring quality in this context demands a different lens: did the patient feel heard? Was suffering addressed holistically? Did their family feel supported? These are outcome variables that matter deeply yet elude easy quantification. AI systems trained on numerical proxies may struggle to recognise when the best outcome is not intervention, but presence.

The danger is not simply that we overlook the intangible, but that we reframe it in ways that distort its meaning. Patient satisfaction surveys, for instance, are often used as stand-ins for experiential quality. But they are fraught with ambiguity—sensitive to mood, expectation, and cultural norms. Moreover, when institutions tie bonuses or penalties to these scores, clinicians may feel pressured to *perform empathy* rather than practice it. *When care becomes a theatre of metrics, authenticity is the casualty.*

There are, of course, efforts to broaden our evaluative frameworks. Initiatives like the Patient-Reported Outcomes Measurement Information System (PROMIS) and Experience-Based Co-Design (EBCD) aim to capture the patient's voice more robustly. But even these risk becoming mechanised if stripped of context. A checkbox labelled "shared decision-making" does not ensure that the conversation was meaningful. A Likert-scale question about emotional support cannot substitute for a real dialogue about fear and uncertainty.

The problem is not with measurement per se, but with *metric monoculture*. When complex realities are reduced to singular scores—be it a risk percentage, a satisfaction index, or a mortality ratio—we lose the granularity that makes care relational and humane. Worse, we risk misallocating attention. A hospital may invest heavily in lowering sepsis mortality through algorithmic alerts, while neglecting the chronic discomfort and isolation of its long-stay elderly patients—because the former is easier to benchmark.

One way forward is to distinguish between *performance metrics* and *meaningful indicators*. The former track compliance with standards; the latter reflect values that matter to patients and communities. For example, rather than merely measuring whether a diabetic patient's HbA1c is under control, we might ask: can the patient maintain their cultural diet without shame? Can they afford their medication without financial distress? These questions open up a richer, value-sensitive form of evaluation.

Such shifts require reimagining what counts as evidence. In community-based mental health services, for instance, traditional metrics often fail to capture progress. A patient may still experience symptoms, but regain the capacity to attend school or re-establish family relationships. These outcomes are real and transformative, but they are also diffuse, co-produced, and context-dependent. *They emerge not from standardised treatments but from trust, time, and tailored engagement.*

Importantly, AI systems can either reinforce or challenge this status quo. If designed narrowly, they will prioritise efficiency and throughput, treating human stories as noise. But if designed ethically, they can incorporate broader definitions of success. For example, natural language processing could help identify themes in patient narratives, surfacing concerns that traditional surveys miss. Machine learning models could be trained not only on survival rates but on *functional recovery*, *social reintegration*, or *values concordance*. These models would require new data sources, new labels, and new kinds of interdisciplinary collaboration—but they would better reflect what patients and clinicians actually care about.

A few pioneering projects already hint at this potential. In the UK, the Health Foundation's work on "Measuring What

Matters" has supported local NHS trusts in developing bespoke outcome sets, co-designed with patients. In Camden, New Jersey, the Camden Coalition uses a "complexity lens" to evaluate interventions not just on cost savings, but on relational continuity, housing stability, and perceived agency. These efforts are messy, contested, and iterative—but they offer a glimpse of a more *democratic epistemology*, where care quality is not imposed from above but defined from within.

There is also a need to recognise the role of clinicians as epistemic agents. When quality is measured solely through documentation and data entry, their moral and interpretive labour is devalued. A good GP knows that a patient's tone of voice, a spouse's body language, or a long pause before answering a question may reveal more than the blood test just received. But these clues do not register in the system. Worse, the time taken to attend to them may be punished under productivity metrics. *The art of noticing becomes a liability.*

To protect this form of professional judgement, evaluative systems must include *narrative capture*, *case reflection*, and *peer dialogue* as legitimate tools of assessment. This is not nostalgia for a pre-digital age, but a recognition that some truths reside in stories, not spreadsheets. Moreover, inviting patients and professionals to interpret outcomes together—through feedback loops, collaborative audits, or narrative reviews—rebuilds trust. It reframes evaluation as shared meaning-making rather than external policing.

Of course, such approaches demand a tolerance for ambiguity. They resist the lure of tidy dashboards and league tables. But that is the point. Healthcare is not a factory. It is a moral practice conducted under conditions of uncertainty. *To pretend otherwise is not scientific rigour; it is bureaucratic delusion.*

Ultimately, we must ask: *What kind of healthcare do we want to build?* One that optimises for what is easy to count—or one that attends to what matters most? The answer requires courage, not just coding. It requires that we hold space for nuance, listen across difference, and develop evaluative tools that honour the full spectrum of care.

Metrics will always have their place. But they must serve as *a compass, not a cage*. When we centre meaning over measurement, we reclaim healthcare as a human endeavour—not just a system to be monitored, but a relationship to be stewarded. Only then can we say with confidence that we are measuring what truly matters.

Chapter 8
Health in Cultural Context

A patient presents with chronic pain. She is a Black woman in her thirties. Her vital signs fall within normal ranges; imaging yields no conclusive results. The AI-assisted triage system slots her into a low-risk queue. Objectively, efficiently, the algorithm has performed its function. Yet beneath this apparent neutrality lies a persistent shadow: decades of research show that Black women are systematically undertreated for pain. Here, the machine did not choose to discriminate—it inherited discrimination. Algorithmic bias often begins in the data, and that data begins in human observation: the world interprets certain bodies not as they are, but as it has learned to perceive them.

This is the unsettling truth at the heart of modern healthcare's embrace of AI: the illusion of neutrality masks deeply ingrained patterns of cultural assumption, institutional precedent, and sociotechnical design. Far from existing outside prejudice, AI can amplify it. Deployed at scale—through diagnostic aids, triage prioritisation, or personalised care recommendations—these systems do more than mediate decisions. They mediate whose symptoms are believed, whose suffering is legible, whose lives are acknowledged within the clinical gaze. The body is never purely biological; it is simultaneously a social signal, a cultural text, a site where data and meaning collide.

Those most vulnerable are often those whose experiences are already marginalised in clinical frameworks. A non-verbal autistic teenager. A transgender man with abdominal pain. A rural woman with limited internet access. Their presentations may lie outside the datasets that train most models—not because their experiences are rare, but because the recording of their experiences has historically been incomplete or biased. Absence in data is never a mere technical oversight; it is a symptom of structural erasure.

Western medical epistemology—the foundation of most health AI—privileges objectivity, linear causality, and reductionist biology. This has enabled enormous advances, yet it is not universal. In many cultural contexts, health is relational, spiritual, or ecological; symptoms may be conveyed metaphorically, communally, or through ritual. Traditional systems of medicine—from Ayurveda to Indigenous healing—value narrative and context in ways resistant to digitisation. When Western AI models are applied globally, these rich interpretive frameworks are often dismissed as noise or anomaly. The result is not simply a loss of nuance—it is an erosion of sovereignty.

Global health AI carries the risk of quiet epistemic imperialism. Consider diagnostic tools deployed in low-resource regions of the Global South. The promise is real: faster triage, early detection, scalable care. But whose norms guide these designs? Whose bodies populate the datasets? Whose understandings of health, illness, and acceptable risk are encoded? Without culturally embedded design, these tools risk reproducing a colonial logic: local patients made legible only through external paradigms, traditional healers sidelined, indigenous knowledge overwritten by statistical abstraction. Technology that arrives without listening is a monologue, not a dialogue.

The challenge is not merely technical. It is ethical, political, and epistemic. Can AI respect pluralistic health paradigms? Can it attend to difference without flattening it into deviation? This requires more than diverse data; it demands rethinking the categorisation of knowledge, the validation of voices, and the translation of cultural nuance into computationally actionable forms. Cultural competence in code is not a checklist—it is an orientation, one that embraces specificity over universality.

Some innovators are taking this seriously. Participatory algorithm design, community-led data annotation, and culturally grounded interface testing offer glimpses of a more equitable future. In South Africa, HIV care apps co-designed with patients and community health workers embed local idioms, values, and decision-making protocols. In Canada, Indigenous-led research guides AI developers in incorporating collective data governance and traditional knowledge frameworks. These are not mere case studies—they are proof that alternative pathways exist.

Narrative has always been a form of resistance. For communities historically misrepresented in biomedical records, stories—oral histories, community health archives—preserve not just facts, but frames: who gets to speak, how illness is understood, what counts as evidence. Within AI, these narratives act as a counterweight, reminding us that datasets freeze the past, and without intervention, tomorrow's tools may entrench yesterday's injustices. Stories assert the patient as narrator, not merely as subject.

Narrative also offers a lens for evaluation. Beyond accuracy metrics and deployment efficiency lies a deeper question: Do AI tools recognise patients as situated beings, with histories, beliefs, and communities? Culturally attuned design is more than bias correction—it is a practice of respect. It asks not just "Does it work?" but "For whom? In what context? At what cost to dignity?"

This chapter situates health AI within a wider contest over meaning, voice, and legitimacy. These are not hypothetical concerns—they are real, everyday design decisions: in data labs, clinical protocols, product meetings, funding allocations. Their outcomes determine who is heard, who receives care, and who is overlooked. Cultural integration is not a postscript to innovation—it is foundational to ethical healthcare in a pluralistic world.

The following discussion offers provocations rather than prescriptions: an invitation to view AI as a site of negotiation. Between global and local. Between standardisation and story. Between efficiency and empathy. Between what can be measured and what must be honoured. Health is culturally situated, and the tools built to protect it must be too. If AI is to serve meaningfully, it must do more than calculate—it must learn to listen.

Not All Bodies Are Interpreted the Same

Two patients walk into the same emergency department, each reporting chest pain. One is a white man in his fifties; the other, a Black woman in her thirties. The first is swiftly routed into a cardiac workup; the second is told to monitor her symptoms and is discharged with a referral for stress management. The decision is not an explicit act of racism. It is the outcome of embedded clinical heuristics—shaped by years of data, practice patterns, and cultural assumptions—quietly reinforced by triage algorithms that learn from historical precedent. *AI did not create the bias; it absorbed it, codified it, and gave it the sheen of objectivity.*

In the context of machine learning, fairness is often framed as a technical problem: How do we remove bias from data? How do we ensure equitable outputs across demographic groups? Yet this framing overlooks a deeper question—*whose experiences are represented, and how are they interpreted*? Algorithms do not encounter symptoms directly. They interpret proxies: biometric signals, electronic records, clinician notes, speech transcripts. Each of these layers is already shaped by human perception—by how pain is described, how disability is documented, how distress is expressed. The illusion of neutrality collapses when we recognise that *data is never raw. It is always cooked in cultural broth*.

Clinical decision support tools trained on large datasets often miss how race, gender, disability, and class shape the expression and reception of symptoms. For example, Black patients have been shown to receive less opioid pain relief for identical injuries compared to white patients, a legacy of debunked theories that falsely claimed Black people have thicker skin or higher pain thresholds. These biases are not confined to individual clinicians—they are reflected in the language of clinical notes, in patterns of medication prescription, and in diagnostic pathways. When AI is trained on this data, it learns a skewed map of human suffering: one in which certain bodies are consistently read as less credible, less urgent, or less worthy of intervention. *What appears as clinical judgment may be, in fact, a systemic failure to see.*

Gender, too, complicates the interpretive machinery of health AI. Women presenting with heart attacks are more likely to be misdiagnosed, in part because their symptoms often differ from the canonical male pattern used to train both physicians and models. Chest pain in men? Urgent. Nausea, fatigue, and jaw pain in women? Vague, psychological, perhaps even hormonal. These differences in presentation are not just medical—they are cultural. Women are socialised to minimise their pain, to avoid seeming hysterical, to accept misdiagnosis as unfortunate but routine. AI, built on this data, learns not to question these silences. It *inherits the gaps without ever knowing they exist.*

Disability introduces another layer of complexity. Consider how electronic health records categorise non-verbal patients, those with cognitive impairments, or individuals with rare syndromes. Standard fields rarely capture nuance; checkbox logic flattens complex lived realities. As a result, these patients often generate outlier data—sparse, inconsistent, nonconforming—which machine learning systems are trained to discount. Outliers are anomalies, and anomalies are filtered out. The very people who most need personalised care become algorithmically invisible. *Their atypicality is treated not as a signal of need, but as statistical noise.*

Socioeconomic status compounds this invisibility. Low-income patients may miss appointments, switch providers frequently, or lack consistent access to digital health tools—all of which can appear to algorithms as disengagement or non-compliance. But these patterns reflect systemic barriers: unstable housing, lack of paid leave, digital illiteracy. When AI systems interpret these data points without social context, they risk making perverse inferences. A patient who cannot afford transportation to the clinic may be labelled high-risk not for her condition, but for her presumed unreliability. *The result is a feedback loop in which social disadvantage is reframed as medical inferiority.*

The challenge is not that AI systems are uniquely biased. It is that they make bias scalable, legible, and harder to contest. Unlike human clinicians, models do not hesitate, justify, or second-guess. Their outputs arrive with the authority of probability—precise, statistical, and often opaque. This can create a chilling effect on dissent. A junior doctor may hesitate to override a model's recommendation, even when it contradicts their intuition. A patient's insistence on their symptoms may be dismissed as noncompliance, especially if the model offers a confident counterdiagnosis. *The algorithm becomes the arbiter of credibility, even when it has no understanding of context.*

To respond effectively, we must rethink what counts as "data" in clinical AI. Structured fields and numeric values are not enough. We need models trained to recognise variation in expression, to attend to the social determinants of health, and to privilege interpretive humility over predictive certainty. Some promising approaches include natural language processing systems that track linguistic markers of distress across different dialects, machine learning models designed to flag diagnostic uncertainty rather than suppress it, and collaborative annotation projects that include patients and community advocates in shaping training datasets. These are not technical tweaks—they are philosophical commitments. *They reflect a view of health data not as a neutral input, but as a cultural artefact.*

Moreover, the design of interfaces matters. When clinicians are presented with risk scores or diagnostic suggestions, the way that information is framed can reinforce or disrupt bias. Does the model display uncertainty? Does it include contextual data—housing instability, caregiver availability, cultural background? Does it allow for annotation, contestation, or patient input? A dashboard that flattens patients into risk categories without room for narrative is not just inadequate. It is dangerous. *Every interface is an ethics interface.*

There is no singular solution to the disparities baked into health data. But there are practices—of listening, contextualising, designing—that can mitigate harm. These begin with a refusal to treat the model as final, and a commitment to keep patients in the loop as narrators of their own experiences. They require clinicians to recognise when their own training has taught them to doubt some patients more than others. And they demand of technologists a broader humility: that prediction without interpretation is not intelligence, but automation in disguise.

Ultimately, *not all bodies are interpreted the same*—not by doctors, not by data, and not by machines. But recognising this asymmetry is the first step toward building systems that honour the full spectrum of human variation. In doing so, we do not merely correct for bias. We create space for dignity.

The Globalization of a Western Model

A diagnostic algorithm trained in Boston evaluates a patient in Nairobi. It flags the case as atypical. The patient has tuberculosis, but the presentation doesn't align with the training data. The model has never seen this combination of symptoms before. Not because it is medically implausible—but because it is geographically and culturally unfamiliar. What the model reads as noise may, in fact, be normal. What it elevates as relevant may be marginal in the local context. *In its logic, efficiency equals familiarity—and familiarity is Western.*

Artificial intelligence in healthcare promises scalability, speed, and predictive precision. But as these systems are exported across borders, they often carry more than their technical capabilities. Embedded within their architecture are the clinical norms, ethical priorities, institutional structures, and cultural assumptions of the environments in which they were built—most often, North America and Western Europe. These biases are not malicious; they are infrastructural. But the consequences are profound. *When AI crosses borders without context, it becomes less a tool for care and more a conduit for epistemic imperialism.*

Consider the global rollout of image-based diagnostic tools for dermatology. Many of the most celebrated models were trained primarily on datasets composed of light-skinned individuals. When these tools are deployed in regions where darker skin tones predominate—across sub-Saharan Africa, South Asia, Latin America—they exhibit markedly lower accuracy. This is not a flaw in the underlying algorithm; it is a failure of imagination in dataset construction. The question isn't whether the model works. It's *for whom* it was built to work. A system that performs with 95% accuracy on European skin types and 65% elsewhere cannot claim universality. It is a parochial intelligence dressed in global clothes.

Language processing systems face similar challenges. Clinical notes in the United States often follow a templated, billing-driven structure: HPI, ROS, PMH, medications. These formats inform natural language processing models that learn to extract diagnoses, detect symptoms, or predict deterioration. But such documentation habits are not global norms. In Brazil, for instance, patient records are often narrative and unstructured. In India, they may be multilingual or handwritten. When AI systems trained on one style of recordkeeping are deployed in another, their performance deteriorates—or worse, they misclassify entirely. The systems don't merely fail to understand. They silently *overwrite* the local grammar of care.

At the level of ethics, the problem deepens. Western healthcare systems tend to centre autonomy, individual consent, and privacy as paramount values. In contrast, many non-Western traditions privilege communal decision-making, interdependence, and spiritual framing of illness. For example, in parts of rural Kenya, decisions about end-of-life care are not made solely by the patient but involve extended family and village elders. A machine-learning model optimised for "patient-centred outcomes" may interpret this as noncompliance, or simply lack the schema to process such dynamics. *What the model calls a deviation may be, locally, the moral centre of care.*

The tension becomes particularly evident when global health initiatives implement predictive models for resource allocation. A triage algorithm designed in the UK and deployed in Southeast Asia may prioritise cases based on standardised metrics like vital signs or laboratory values. But in low-resource settings, such measurements may be unavailable, delayed, or contextually irrelevant. A child's likelihood of survival from sepsis in a Dhaka slum may depend more on proximity to a working ambulance or the availability of family caregivers than on their blood pressure. These are not variables typically found in high-income country datasets. *The algorithm knows what it knows. It does not know what it does not know.*

Some may argue that models can simply be retrained on local data. But this solution assumes that such data is both available and epistemically compatible. In many low-income settings, health records are incomplete, non-digitised, or heavily biased by underreporting. Moreover, the very act of framing health phenomena through Western taxonomies—ICD codes, SNOMED vocabularies, standardised ontologies—can displace local knowledge. Traditional healing practices, informal care networks, and culturally embedded understandings of illness often have no field in the database. The risk is not merely of technical mismatch. It is of *epistemic erasure*—a quiet colonisation of what counts as real, valid, and legible.

This dynamic is particularly visible in mental health. Western models often pathologise distress through diagnostic categories like depression, anxiety, or PTSD. But in many cultures, psychological suffering is expressed somatically or spiritually. In Chinese medicine, for instance, emotions are closely tied to organ systems. In some Indigenous communities in Australia and Canada, wellbeing is inseparable from land, ancestry, and ritual. When AI-based mental health screening tools are trained on Western clinical language, they fail to capture these nuances. Worse, they may *medicalise cultural expression*, interpreting it as disorder rather than difference.

There are, of course, efforts to resist this dynamic. In India, the Aravind Eye Care System has developed its own AI diagnostic tools for cataracts and retinal disease, trained specifically on Indian populations. In Rwanda, local data scientists have worked to develop malaria prediction models using indigenous data sources, rather than importing European tools. These projects are not merely technical adaptations—they represent a shift in authorship, a reclaiming of the right to define what constitutes "normal," "urgent," or "pathological" within a given context.

Yet these local initiatives are exceptions. The prevailing global pipeline still runs in one direction: from Silicon Valley to the Global South; from well-funded hospitals in London to overstretched clinics in Lagos. The deployment is often framed as "capacity building," "knowledge transfer," or "tech for good." But without reciprocal learning, shared authorship, and contextual humility, such efforts risk reproducing the very asymmetries they claim to redress. *When knowledge flows only one way, what is transferred is not just technology—it is hierarchy.*

To avoid this, the global health AI community must interrogate its own assumptions. Whose bodies populate the training sets? Whose definitions of health and illness are encoded in the models? Who gets to decide what counts as ground truth? These are not peripheral questions—they are foundational. An algorithm cannot be culturally neutral if its development process is not. A model cannot be globally applicable if its logic excludes the majority of the world's healthcare realities.

This does not mean abandoning AI in global health. It means designing with difference in mind. It means funding projects led by local researchers, clinicians, and patients. It means building infrastructures that accommodate pluralism rather than demanding conformity. And it means recognising that *imported intelligence, however sophisticated, is no substitute for contextual wisdom.*

Ultimately, the promise of AI in healthcare will be measured not by how efficiently it replicates Western standards, but by how effectively it respects and responds to local meaning. This requires more than technical refinement. It demands a political and ethical shift: from exporting solutions to *sharing stewardship*. Only then can global health AI move from a colonial inheritance to a truly collaborative future.

Cultural Competence in Code

In clinical settings, cultural competence once referred to a physician's ability to listen without bias, communicate across difference, and tailor care to patients' backgrounds. Today, as algorithmic systems enter the exam room, the definition demands an update. Can a model trained on Western symptom vocabularies understand grief in rural Ethiopia, where bereavement is not a clinical event but a community ritual? Can a triage algorithm account for how Somali women describe pain, or why an Indigenous patient might refuse to make eye contact—not out of evasiveness, but respect? These are not semantic footnotes. *They are essential to the ethics and efficacy of care.* And they prompt a question long neglected in the development of healthcare AI: *Can cultural competence be coded?* And if so, *should it?*

The first challenge is architectural. AI models learn from data—volumes of it. But data, especially in healthcare, is not a passive imprint of the world. It is shaped by what gets recorded, by whom, and for what purpose. Consider electronic health records (EHRs). In high-income countries, most clinical interactions are documented digitally, driven by insurance codes, billing incentives, and institutional standards. These notes reflect the clinical priorities of their ecosystem. Yet even within such datasets, diversity is often underrepresented. The language of Black patients is more likely to be flagged as "noncompliant," while symptom reports from women are more frequently labelled "anxious" or "psychosomatic." When machine-learning systems are trained on these records, they inherit not only statistical patterns but historical inequities. *Cultural difference is not simply excluded—it is systemically misclassified.*

Beyond representation, there is the problem of expression. Culture shapes how illness is named, interpreted, and prioritised. A sore throat in one context is a trivial nuisance; in another, it is a feared precursor to rheumatic fever. In the

Philippines, the concept of *"ginhawa"* captures a holistic sense of well-being that includes spiritual, social, and physical dimensions. No ICD code can capture this. Yet when AI models reduce health to discrete symptoms and quantifiable metrics, they flatten such complexity. The issue isn't just accuracy—it's *ontology. Whose version of reality is legible to the system?*

Consider natural language processing (NLP) in clinical settings. These systems aim to extract insights from physicians' notes, patient surveys, or telehealth transcripts. But what happens when patients speak in dialects, mix languages, or use idioms unfamiliar to standard lexicons? In Singapore, it's common for patients to blend English, Mandarin, Malay, and Tamil in a single consultation. In Nigeria, patients may describe mental distress through spiritual or familial metaphors. A culturally naive NLP system may misread these as noise or ignore them entirely. Worse, it may make decisions based on misinterpretation, codifying misunderstanding as clinical fact. *When meaning is lost in translation, so is safety.*

This raises a deeper design question. Should we build AI systems that aim to be universally competent, absorbing cultural variance into a grand, global model? Or should we pursue pluralistic architectures—smaller, community-specific models that reflect local norms and practices? The former promises scalability but risks erasure; the latter honours context but complicates interoperability. The ethical calculus is not trivial. A model that generalises across cultures may appear fair in aggregate but fail the individuals it purports to serve. Conversely, a system that reflects the worldview of a specific group may struggle to operate outside it. *There is no neutral ground. Every design decision is a political choice.*

One approach is the development of modular AI systems with culturally adaptable components. Instead of a monolithic model, designers can create frameworks where cultural logic is parameterised—allowing systems to adjust clinical reasoning pathways based on the patient's background. For example, a symptom-checker might weigh family history differently in cultures where intergenerational illness is stigmatised and underreported. Or it might adjust risk communication strategies in communities where fatalism shapes health-seeking behaviour. This requires more than translation; it demands *transcreation*—reimagining the system's logic through a culturally specific lens.

But achieving this level of nuance necessitates inclusive collaboration. The old model—engineers build, clinicians validate, patients comply—is no longer tenable. Developing culturally competent AI requires the epistemic labour of community members, anthropologists, linguistic experts, local health workers, and patients themselves. Their insights are not add-ons; they are infrastructural. In Maori communities, for example, researchers have worked with tribal elders to develop digital health tools that honour *whānau* (extended family) structures and spiritual cosmologies. These are not mere cultural wrappers on Western tech—they are *conceptual reorientations* of what health means.

Yet this kind of co-creation poses a challenge to conventional AI development pipelines, which are optimised for efficiency, not deliberation. Training a culturally nuanced model takes longer, costs more, and requires a willingness to entertain ambiguity. Data must be cleaned, annotated, and interpreted with attention to local meaning. Statistical anomalies must be investigated, not discarded. Outliers may be signals of cultural variance, not noise. For most commercial entities, this level of granularity is viewed as a liability. But for ethical design, it is essential. *Speed is not the enemy of care—but uniformity might be.*

Critics argue that cultural competence in AI is an unattainable ideal. Human clinicians, after all, struggle with cultural bias despite years of training. How can machines, built from abstractions and correlations, do better? But this objection misunderstands the goal. The aim is not to encode perfect understanding, but to *design for humility*. A culturally competent system does not claim to know all things; it knows what it does not know. It flags uncertainty, invites human oversight, and creates space for dialogue rather than dictation. It is less a seer than a steward—a tool for negotiation rather than enforcement.

This reframing requires a shift in how we evaluate AI performance. Standard metrics—accuracy, sensitivity, specificity—are necessary but insufficient. We must also measure interpretability, trustworthiness, and cultural resonance. Does the system foster dignity in patient interactions? Does it support clinicians in understanding, not overriding, cultural context? Does it make visible the limits of its own competence? These are not philosophical luxuries. They are *design imperatives*, especially in multicultural health environments.

Some institutions are beginning to take this seriously. The WHO has convened working groups on ethical AI in global health that include cultural considerations. Initiatives like Datasphere and AI4D Africa are funding projects that build locally grounded data ecosystems. In the U.S., the Office of the National Coordinator for Health IT has issued guidelines that include equity and cultural responsiveness in health tech evaluation. But these efforts remain fragmented. There is no consensus standard, no widely adopted toolkit for encoding cultural competence into code. The field is still in its infancy—and the stakes are rising.

Because the alternative is not neutrality. It is automation without reflection. When cultural nuance is absent from AI design, systems do not operate impartially—they operate *ignorantly*. They replicate the perspective of their creators, often unknowingly. And in a domain as intimate and high-stakes as healthcare, that ignorance can harm. *To be blind to culture is not to be objective. It is to be dangerously narrow.*

Cultural competence in AI is not about perfection. It is about participation. It invites us to expand who gets to define health, whose experiences are deemed valid, and how knowledge is translated into action. It requires that we treat cultural variance not as a barrier to be standardised away, but as *a source of design intelligence*. In doing so, we begin to shift the locus of innovation—from algorithmic prowess to *contextual wisdom*.

The future of healthcare AI will not be judged solely by its predictive power, but by its capacity to listen, adapt, and respect. Cultural competence is not a feature to be toggled on; it is a foundational ethic. It shapes how we build, whom we serve, and what kind of care we consider worthy of automation. And it reminds us, urgently, that *what we design reflects what we value*.

Story as Resistance

In a world increasingly shaped by metrics, dashboards, and data pipelines, the human voice is too often reduced to a data point—quantifiable, sortable, and stripped of narrative context. In healthcare, this abstraction is not benign. When a patient's story is collapsed into symptom codes and probability weights, what is lost is not merely nuance, but personhood. *Narrative resists this flattening.* It insists that health is not merely a collection of signs and numbers but an unfolding, lived experience. Where artificial intelligence favours scale, speed, and uniformity, story moves slowly, situated in time, place, and relation. And in doing so, it becomes a form of cultural resistance—a way communities reclaim agency against systems that mistake prediction for understanding.

The rise of AI in medicine has amplified a longstanding tension between standardisation and subjectivity. Clinical guidelines and decision trees were designed to reduce error and promote evidence-based care. Yet these frameworks often presume universality where there is diversity, and linearity where there is complexity. AI systems, trained on such paradigms, intensify the pattern: patients are routed through model pathways that optimise for outcomes defined not by the patient, but by statistical models. In this regime, *stories are inconvenient.* They introduce uncertainty. They disrupt the logic of automation. They force us to pause.

And yet it is in this pause that meaning resides. Consider a case from northern Canada, where Indigenous health workers have long used "healing circles" to support those experiencing depression and trauma. These gatherings are not therapy in the Western clinical sense; they are oral traditions that blend storytelling, shared memory, ritual, and communal witnessing. They resist the reduction of suffering to pathology. When digital mental health tools were introduced to the region—apps built to deliver CBT (Cognitive Behavioural Therapy) interventions—engagement was low. Not because the tools were poorly designed technically, but because they spoke a different language. *They offered strategies where people wanted stories.* Community health leaders responded not by rejecting technology, but by reshaping it—embedding Indigenous narratives into digital formats that honoured local cosmologies of care. *Story, in this context, was not nostalgic—it was adaptive.*

The power of narrative lies not only in what it conveys but in what it makes possible. Stories carry moral weight. They transmit values, social roles, and historical memory. In many cultures, especially those whose knowledge systems were marginalised by colonial medicine, stories are epistemologies—they are how knowledge is stored, validated, and passed on. To exclude narrative from AI training datasets is to erase this way of knowing. To insist on structured fields and response formats is to impose a logic that privileges certain ways of being ill, of seeking help, of making sense. *The danger is not only exclusion—it is epistemic violence.*

In urban hospitals, the tension is equally present, if more subtly encoded. A patient from a working-class background, describing fatigue, financial stress, and chronic pain in a stream-of-consciousness style, may be dismissed as unfocused or noncompliant. A more affluent patient, describing similar issues in medicalised language, may receive prompt follow-up and compassionate engagement. When AI systems are trained on clinician notes that reflect these biases, they begin to learn not only what symptoms matter, but *whose voice counts*. They may learn that Black patients' pain reports are less reliable. That women's cardiac symptoms are less urgent. That mental health crises among undocumented migrants are behavioural, not medical. These are not algorithmic failures; they are *systemic biases encoded in the absence of story*.

Some researchers argue that narrative is simply too difficult to process at scale—that AI needs structure, standardisation, and consistency to function. But this objection underestimates what is technologically possible and philosophically necessary. Natural language processing (NLP) systems, for example, can now capture sentiment, metaphor, temporal relationships, and contextual ambiguity. The problem is not technological incapacity, but institutional priorities. Most AI systems are built to optimise for billing, compliance, or throughput—not for meaning, dignity, or connection. *We have chosen metrics over meaning—not because it is easier, but because it is more profitable.*

Yet around the world, countercurrents are forming. In Brazil, public health workers in the favelas have developed mobile apps that allow community members to record health stories in their own words—voice notes that capture not only symptoms, but context. These narratives are reviewed by local health agents who know the families, the history, the terrain. AI is used not to interpret the stories directly, but to detect patterns and surface prompts for deeper human engagement. *The machine supports the listener, not the arbiter.* It's an inversion of the typical model—less about prediction, more about presence.

In the United States, palliative care teams have begun integrating life-story interviews into electronic health records. Patients nearing the end of life are invited to reflect on key experiences, relationships, and values. These narratives are summarised—not algorithmically, but by human staff—and placed at the top of the clinical chart. When decisions are being made about pain management, life support, or discharge planning, the patient's voice is not inferred; it is present. The stories do not replace medical data, but *reframe what matters.* AI systems that engage with such records are thus trained not only on outcomes, but on meaning.

Even in high-tech environments, the absence of story is beginning to be felt. In Silicon Valley, several prominent hospitals have adopted AI scribes—digital assistants that transcribe and summarise doctor-patient conversations. Initially hailed as time-saving breakthroughs, many clinicians report that they feel more alienated than ever. The summarised notes often miss key emotional cues, flatten patient language, or strip context. Some doctors have begun annotating the summaries manually, reintroducing nuance. Others are calling for design changes—prompting the AI to flag ambiguity, emotional tone, or patient narratives that diverge from expected trajectories. The lesson is clear: *systems that ignore story must be corrected by humans who remember its value.*

This is not an argument against AI in healthcare. It is an argument against amnesia. Against the forgetting of traditions—whether Indigenous or working-class, immigrant or ancestral—that carry health knowledge through story. Against the false belief that data is neutral, and that standardisation is synonymous with fairness. Against the quiet violence of abstraction, where people become profiles, and pain becomes a percentage.

Narrative resists because it remembers. It insists that every body has a context. That health is not an equation but a relationship. That suffering is not always a problem to be solved, but sometimes a truth to be witnessed. And it offers a challenge to designers, policymakers, and clinicians alike: *Will you make space for the story?* Not as a cosmetic feature, not as a checkbox for inclusion, but as a foundation for care?

In the end, story is not only what patients tell—it is what communities keep. It is the collective memory of survival, of adaptation, of meaning-making under pressure. In systems that overlook this, resistance is not optional—it is necessary. And it comes not through outrage, but through voice. Through the stories that say: *We are still here. We have our own language for health. And we will not be reduced.*

Chapter 9
Decision Fatigue and the Burden of Choice

Choice, once heralded as the pinnacle of autonomy, now carries a curious ambivalence in modern healthcare. What was meant to empower—the ability to select treatments, navigate platforms, and tailor one's health journey—has often morphed into a source of cognitive burden. Precision medicine promised clarity: more data, more insight, more meaningful decisions. Yet the reality for many patients is the opposite. The proliferation of tailored options rarely liberates; it overwhelms. What should be agency becomes anxiety, as each new pathway hints at a "better" alternative, leaving patients unsettled and second-guessing. This chapter opens with that tension: the uneasy terrain where autonomy and exhaustion meet.

Today's patient is asked to be more than recipient; they are co-analyst, co-designer, co-decider. They weigh treatment protocols, side-effect projections, and competing algorithmic forecasts—all while navigating pain, urgency, or emotional strain. What once might have been a relatively linear sequence—describe symptoms, receive diagnosis, follow plan—now unfurls through dashboards, probabilistic models, and risk stratifications. Customisation, celebrated as empowerment, often becomes the labour of managing the management of illness itself. The patient is not merely ill; they are responsible for curating their own care.

This is not simply a matter of interface design. The ethos of optimisation permeates contemporary healthcare. Every choice seems subject to fine-tuning. Yet when every path is provisional, constantly recalculated by data streams and predictive engines, the pursuit of "perfect care" can feel like a relentless audit. A cancer patient, for instance, may confront eight genomic-targeted therapy regimens, each accompanied by app-generated forecasts of side effects, quality-of-life projections, and cohort-based outcomes. Every hesitation, every click, becomes traceable, potentially feeding back into optimisation algorithms. In this context, choice is not merely empowered; it is surveilled.

The culture of continual optimisation reshapes expectations as much as experiences. Patients—and indeed even the healthy—internalise the logic that there is always a better sleep, a more efficient glucose monitor, a more optimised diet. Illness is reframed as a performance deficit; health is an achievement demanding constant vigilance. Daily acts—eating, walking, sleeping—become programmable behaviours, subject to metrics and refinement. The patient assumes perpetual custodianship of their own wellness, and health becomes an elusive, moving target.

Beneath this lies a deeper ethical question: who decides what merits optimisation? AI systems rarely function as neutral arbiters. Algorithms reflect institutional priorities, economic incentives, and historical data shaped by social inequities. A triage model may optimise throughput at the expense of rare presentations. A diagnostic tool may favour common pathologies, neglecting low-incidence but high-impact conditions. Even apps designed for adherence embed invisible norms and values, often distant from the patient's lived context. What the system "recommends" is not just statistically likely—it is what someone somewhere has deemed desirable.

Here emerges the need for epistemic humility. Are these systems genuinely supporting decision-making, or subtly coercing it? How confident can patients—or clinicians—be in resisting algorithmic guidance without fear of being labelled noncompliant? In traditional practice, a physician might say,

"There's no single correct path; let's explore options." In AI-mediated care, pluralism flattens under probability-weighted decision paths. Deviating from the recommended course can feel reckless; uncertainty, an essential aspect of medicine, is treated as an error to be corrected.

Yet uncertainty is not failure—it is the index of complexity. Illness unfolds across bodies, histories, relationships, and emotions that no model can fully capture. Systems that claim a "God view," assuming that all variables can be measured, risk rendering invisible the subtle textures of lived experience. The consequence is cognitive overload and moral disorientation. Patients may defer to systems that make algorithmic sense but feel intuitively wrong—not from ignorance, but from diminished trust in their own judgment.

The remedy is not sleeker interfaces or prettier visualisations. It is a reorientation of design: away from optimisation-as-default and toward support for ambiguity. Tools should acknowledge complexity without rushing to resolve it. Decision aids can present trade-offs rather than directives, allowing patients space to pause, reflect, and even reject recommendations without penalty. This is not anti-technology—it is human-centred design at its most ethical, recognising cognition as finite, emotions as valid, and meaning as irreducible.

Some signs of this shift exist. Paediatric oncology units, for instance, are experimenting with "shared decision-making dashboards" that visualise care options not by predicted success alone, but by the values each choice reflects: survival, family time, side-effect burden, school reintegration. In behavioural health, AI-driven apps prompt patients to prioritise what matters most—stability, relationships, autonomy—and adjust guidance accordingly. These are small interventions, but significant ones: they recognise that health is always more than measurable metrics.

Ultimately, this reflection is not a denunciation of technology, but an appeal to reimagine its role. AI in healthcare should aspire not to omniscience, but to companionship. It should not demand decisiveness, but nurture deliberation. It should not feign certainty, but scaffold confidence. If choice is to be meaningful, clarity must accompany it—not merely in data, but in the ethics of presentation. Care, after all, exists in the space where information meets understanding, and where human fallibility is respected.

This chapter invites readers to interrogate the architectures of modern healthcare: the tools, the ideologies, the design assumptions that shape patient experience. It asks whether current systems support what it means to be human—fallible, feeling, uncertain, yet capable of judgment. And it reminds us, sometimes, that the wisest choice is the one not made immediately.

Personalisation as Cognitive Overload

There is a curious irony embedded in the promise of AI-enabled personalisation in healthcare. Designed ostensibly to restore patient agency and optimise medical decisions to individual needs, such systems often deliver the opposite: paralysis by abundance. What was once heralded as liberation from generalised care is fast becoming a labyrinth of choices that patients are neither prepared for nor supported in navigating. *The very tools meant to tailor care are, paradoxically, burdening patients with decisions they are neither clinically qualified nor emotionally equipped to make.*

Much of modern medicine's momentum has been defined by a transition from paternalism to autonomy—an overdue correction to centuries of medical authority dictating patient experience. Yet in digital health environments, autonomy has morphed into an expectation of micro-decision-making. Platforms offer dozens of "paths" based on symptoms, genetic data, lifestyle logs, wearable outputs, or behavioural inferences. Choose your risk tolerance. Choose your preferred balance of side effects. Choose whether to prioritise speed, cost, comfort, or evidence. But do so in the absence of consistent human guidance, and often without understanding the full implications of each fork in the road. This is not agency. *It is administrative labour cloaked in the rhetoric of empowerment.*

To understand the burden imposed by personalisation, we must first interrogate how healthcare systems conceive of choice. In consumer logic, more choice equals more value. In clinical logic, the opposite often holds. For most patients—especially those facing serious or chronic conditions—what is needed is not a menu but a compass. *Health decisions are not preference shopping; they are high-stakes judgments made under stress, uncertainty, and asymmetry of information.* When platforms attempt to flatten this complexity into "smart" recommendation interfaces, they often misread the role of context, intuition, and trust in medical decision-making.

Consider the experience of patients managing chronic conditions like diabetes or autoimmune disease. Many digital platforms now offer daily or even hourly recommendations: adjust your insulin based on this projected blood sugar curve; tweak your diet based on sleep patterns; reorder your medication based on activity levels. These micro-optimisations may be statistically defensible, but they create *a condition of continual deliberation*. Instead of freeing patients to live their lives, personalisation can trap them in a state of low-grade vigilance—constantly weighing options, questioning defaults, and second-guessing themselves. The emotional tax of this cognitive engagement is rarely discussed in clinical trials or design briefs. But it is profoundly real.

Clinicians, too, are affected. AI-powered decision support tools routinely bombard doctors with a matrix of options derived from algorithms trained on population data, patient history, and real-time diagnostics. While these tools promise objectivity, they also complicate the process of clinical judgment. Should the physician trust the model's highest-ranked option, or defer to their own diagnostic intuition? Should they relay every potential pathway to the patient, even those marginally less likely to succeed? In an environment where deviation from algorithmic guidance must be justified, *decision-making becomes defensive, not collaborative.* Time that could be spent on meaningful dialogue is instead swallowed by the need to manage options—many of which are designed to check liability boxes rather than support human reasoning.

The psychological toll of excessive choice is not unique to healthcare, but its consequences here are far more severe. Research in behavioural economics has long shown that too many options can lead to decision fatigue, increased regret, and even outright avoidance. In medicine, the stakes are life-altering. Patients overwhelmed by decision complexity may delay care, opt for default recommendations regardless of personal fit, or disengage entirely. Personalisation, when poorly implemented, does not enable better decisions—it sabotages them.

There is also a deeper philosophical tension at play. AI systems operate on a logic of optimisation: more data, better predictions, narrower tailoring. But *what constitutes "better" is rarely neutral.* Personalisation algorithms are calibrated against metrics defined by researchers, insurers, or developers—adherence, cost-efficiency, population risk reduction. These may not align with what a particular patient values: stability over novelty, dignity over duration, quality over quantity. When platforms offer "choices," they do so from a pre-curated universe shaped by these underlying priorities. The patient's voice is not absent, but it is already constrained.

Cultural and socioeconomic disparities compound the issue. Personalisation assumes that patients have the literacy, confidence, and bandwidth to navigate options with discernment. But this is not a given. Marginalised patients, or those with limited English proficiency, cognitive impairment, or low health literacy, face additional burdens. The more "intelligent" the system, the more it may presume a level of interaction fluency that excludes precisely those who most need support. What is pitched as an equitable advancement risks becoming yet another axis of stratification. *A personalised interface is not inherently inclusive—it is only as just as the assumptions built into it.*

Some designers have begun to push back against this overload model. One promising approach involves *adaptive simplicity*: interfaces that initially present only the most clinically appropriate choice, then progressively disclose alternatives based on patient curiosity or hesitation. This preserves autonomy without imposing it as a default burden. Another strategy is *conversational design*—embedding AI systems within guided dialogues that mimic the cadence and empathy of a clinical conversation rather than a product catalogue. These approaches treat patients not as end-users to be optimised, but as partners in a meaning-making process.

Still, these remain exceptions. The prevailing trend continues to valorise granularity: more data, more nuance, more segmentation. The problem is not that tailoring is inherently bad, but that it too often assumes patients want to become their own care architects. Many do not. They want to be seen, heard, understood, and advised. Not nudged, tiered, routed, or rendered into variables. *Personalisation should not mean handing over a complex control panel—it should mean offering a stable hand on the wheel.*

If we are to salvage the promise of personalisation, it must be reoriented away from choice for its own sake. What matters is not how many options a patient is given, but how thoughtfully those options are mediated—by clinicians, by context, and by systems that prioritise clarity over complexity. Only then can personalisation become truly humane: not an algorithmic display of precision, but *a quiet affirmation that the individual before us matters more than the model behind them.*

The Tyranny of Optimization

Optimisation is the reigning doctrine of our technological age. From logistics networks to dating algorithms, from dietary plans to digital interfaces, we are taught to believe that there is always a better version of ourselves waiting to be unlocked—if only we make the right selections, follow the right metrics, and submit ourselves to the right feedback loops. Nowhere has this logic grown more seductive, or more dangerous, than in the domain of health. The application of artificial intelligence in healthcare has brought remarkable efficiencies and diagnostic advances, but it has also imported an ethic of constant improvement—one that reduces wellbeing to variables, rewards compliance over autonomy, and risks eroding the very meaning of care. The pursuit of the "optimal" has become a tyranny not just because it narrows our understanding of health, but because it insists that anything less than maximised is a failure.

At the heart of this paradigm lies a shift in how we define the goal of medicine. Historically, healthcare sought to restore function, relieve suffering, and respect the bounds of human limitation. Today, it is increasingly framed as a system of perpetual enhancement: extending life expectancy, minimising risk, and calibrating every intervention for maximum output. This shift did not begin with AI, but AI systems—particularly those driven by predictive modelling and behavioural nudging—have accelerated it to a degree once unimaginable. Optimisation algorithms do not merely assist decision-making; they embed within clinical practice a set of assumptions about what counts as valuable, desirable, and acceptable. And these assumptions are not neutral.

Consider how an AI system designed to reduce hospital readmissions may prioritise cost efficiency over patient comfort, or how a recommendation engine might nudge a patient toward a medication that statistically improves a biomarker, without regard for the patient's lived experience of side effects. The logic of optimisation flattens complexity. It functions best when variables can be quantified, goals can be standardised, and outcomes can be ranked. But human health is neither linear nor uniform. To assume that there is always a more optimal state to be achieved is to ignore the richness of individual priorities, cultural contexts, and the fundamentally uncertain nature of bodily life.

This pressure toward optimisation also has profound psychological effects. Patients are increasingly cast as decision-makers in a labyrinth of possibilities, where each choice carries the weight of statistical probabilities and algorithmic judgments. The promise of personalised care can morph into the burden of perfectibility. A patient navigating cancer treatment may be presented with not one, but dozens of "paths," each quantified by survival rates, genetic markers, and treatment response models. The narrative offered by the system is clear: choose wisely, and you may live longer. But choice under such circumstances is not empowering—it is paralysing. The responsibility for outcomes, once held jointly between clinician and patient, now subtly shifts toward the patient, who is expected to optimise their path through an ever-expanding matrix of medical options.

The philosophical underpinnings of this trend are rarely interrogated. Optimisation assumes that more is better—that efficiency, longevity, and measurable gains are inherently good. But this overlooks the trade-offs that real patients face. A life extended by months at the cost of dignity may not be optimal by the values of the person living it. A treatment that boosts clinical scores while eroding quality of life may satisfy a model but betray a patient's deeper needs. And a health system that rewards adherence to protocol over personal context risks converting care into compliance. *The tyranny of optimisation is not just about tools—it is about values smuggled in through metrics.*

It is worth asking: who defines the optimal? AI systems are trained on data—vast, retrospective, and deeply contingent. The patterns they detect are shaped by historical norms, institutional incentives, and clinical conventions that reflect biases as much as biology. If a system is trained on datasets where younger, wealthier, or majority populations are overrepresented, its optimisation targets will favour those groups. The ideal blood pressure, the acceptable pain threshold, the recommended course of action—these are not universal truths, but statistical abstractions. When AI systems convert these into prescriptions, they risk marginalising anyone whose needs or bodies fall outside the training set.

This issue becomes even more pronounced when optimisation feeds into performance-based healthcare systems. Clinicians may feel compelled to follow AI-generated guidelines not because they are right for the patient in front of them, but because deviating from them may flag lower efficiency scores or regulatory risk. The clinician's craft—the ability to negotiate uncertainty, build trust, and respond intuitively to patient nuance—is subordinated to the algorithmic imperative. *The system trains its users to optimise, not to understand.*

Indeed, the very language of health becomes technocratic under optimisation logic. We speak of inputs and outputs, adherence and deviation, signal and noise. Suffering is recast as inefficiency. Healing becomes a matter of system throughput. This is not an argument against the use of metrics or the potential of AI. Rather, it is a call to resist the ideology that assumes that if something can be optimised, it should be. There are dimensions of human health—pain, uncertainty, grief, acceptance—that are not failures to be corrected but conditions to be held with care.

Real-world examples illustrate this tension. A study of diabetic patients using AI-guided glucose monitoring found that while glycaemic control improved, many patients reported increased anxiety, burnout, and social withdrawal. The optimisation of blood sugar metrics came at the cost of psychological wellbeing. Another case involved a cancer screening algorithm that significantly increased early detection—but also led to a surge in unnecessary interventions, with physical and emotional consequences for patients who were overtreated. *What the system deemed "better" outcomes were not experienced as such by those undergoing them.*

The allure of optimisation lies in its simplicity. It offers clear goals, rational pathways, and measurable progress. In a domain as uncertain and emotionally charged as health, this can be deeply comforting. But clarity is not the same as truth. *To optimise without asking "for whom, and at what cost?" is to commit a kind of epistemic violence—silencing the messy, plural, and subjective dimensions of being well.* It is to treat life as a problem to be solved rather than a condition to be lived.

What might it look like to resist this tyranny? It would mean designing AI systems that recognise trade-offs, contextualise recommendations, and respect ambiguity. It would mean creating interfaces that ask patients not only what they want to improve, but what they are willing to endure, forego, or accept. It would mean embedding in our health technologies not just metrics for success, but mechanisms for reflection. A system that respects patient autonomy must make space for imperfection—not because perfection is unreachable, but because it is often irrelevant.

Letting go of the optimisation mindset does not mean surrendering to chaos or abandoning the pursuit of better care. It means reorienting our definitions of better. It means understanding that health is not a destination but a relationship: with our bodies, with our caregivers, and with the limits of control. In this light, AI is not a saviour or a villain, but a mirror—reflecting the values we encode within it. If we insist on seeing health only through the lens of improvement, we will lose sight of what makes it worth having. *Sometimes, the most humane outcome is not the most optimised one.*

Who Decides What Matters?

When a patient sits before a physician, they do so with a story—not merely a set of symptoms. And yet, as artificial intelligence increasingly intermediates clinical decisions, that story is filtered, reframed, and frequently flattened into the statistical. What matters, then, is no longer what the patient values or fears, but what the algorithm has been trained to prioritise. In this transference of power, a critical question emerges—who decides what matters? Not just in the moment of decision, but in the very scaffolding of the system that shapes those decisions.

AI systems do not begin from a tabula rasa. Every machine learning model, regardless of sophistication, is shaped by a set of initial assumptions—by what data is collected, how it is labelled, what outcomes are deemed successful, and which metrics are elevated as targets for optimisation. Efficiency, longevity, and cost-effectiveness often headline these models' objectives. And while these values are not inherently problematic, their elevation to primary status—unchallenged, unexamined—creates a framework of care that subtly but powerfully shifts medicine's moral centre.

Consider the design of hospital readmission prediction models. These tools, widely adopted in the United States and increasingly exported abroad, are trained to identify patients at risk of returning to hospital within a defined period. Their goal is to reduce unnecessary readmissions, thereby saving costs and improving system performance. But the model does not account for whether the readmission was clinically appropriate, emotionally necessary, or socially inevitable. It does not understand whether a patient returned because their pain was dismissed, because their housing was unstable, or because they simply had no one else to turn to. The metric becomes a proxy for quality—yet it may encode, invisibly, an architecture of neglect.

Optimisation presumes clarity of goals. But health is not engineering. It is an evolving conversation between science, culture, and values. What is optimal for one patient may feel hollow or even harmful to another. A terminally ill patient may prioritise a lucid goodbye over another cycle of chemotherapy. A new mother with chronic pain may trade functional mobility for alertness sufficient to breastfeed. These nuances—real, human, inescapably subjective—rarely survive the abstraction process required to feed machine learning models.

This is not an indictment of technology itself, but of a value vacuum. When we design optimisation frameworks in healthcare AI, we are not merely encoding preferences—we are enshrining power. Whose definitions of success are we using? Who sets the benchmark for a life well-lived, a body worth preserving, or a treatment worth enduring? Too often, the answer is a small circle of clinical, commercial, and technical actors—those furthest removed from the lived messiness of patient realities.

Take, for instance, the proliferation of wearable health devices and personalised health apps. These tools promise empowerment—letting users "take control" of their wellness through step counts, sleep scores, heart rate variability, and diet optimisation. But they also usher in a quiet coercion. They nudge users toward a version of health defined by quantification, standardisation, and relentless improvement. A person who walks for pleasure, rests when fatigued, or eats communally rather than nutritionally may be labelled suboptimal—not because they are unwell, but because they are unmeasurable within the tool's epistemology.

This techno-moral tension grows sharper in contexts where cultural difference or historical marginalisation intersect with data-driven systems. In many Indigenous communities, for example, health is understood holistically—intertwined with land, lineage, and ritual. An AI system optimised for individual biometric indicators, disconnected from social or spiritual context, will not only misfire technically but may actively undermine the community's conception of care. Similarly, disability advocates have raised concerns that optimisation for certain "normative" functioning baselines can pathologise bodies that deviate from standard measures, even when those bodies are flourishing by their own criteria.

Efforts to create more inclusive datasets and culturally aware design practices are important. But technical adjustments alone cannot solve a fundamentally ethical challenge. The question of who decides what matters is not just a design flaw—it is a governance issue. It calls for deliberation, plurality, and humility. It requires that we ask not only what works, but for whom, under what conditions, and with what trade-offs.

Some promising examples suggest what this might look like in practice. In community-led health initiatives in Kenya, AI tools for maternal health monitoring are co-developed with local midwives, ensuring that predictive alerts are balanced by cultural knowledge and local trust networks. In Norway, participatory data governance models have given Sámi communities a direct role in defining what kinds of data are collected and how they are interpreted. These are not just technocratic tweaks—they are power redistributions.

Even within high-tech hospital systems, there are ways to interrogate optimisation logic. Clinicians at some US academic medical centres are beginning to work with ethicists and patient advisory councils to audit AI models—not just for accuracy, but for alignment with patient values. A predictive tool for ICU triage might be technically sound, but if it systematically deprioritises elderly patients based on survival odds alone, is it just? Is it caring? Is it humane?

This kind of reflective design requires more than ethics checklists or regulatory compliance. It demands philosophical rigour and democratic engagement. It calls on us to remember that care is not a computation problem to be solved, but a relationship to be stewarded. That no model, however elegant, can fully predict what matters to a human being navigating vulnerability.

The stakes are high. As AI becomes embedded not only in decision support but in diagnostic pathways, therapy planning, and mental health triage, the values it encodes will shape the scaffolding of care itself. If we fail to interrogate those values, we risk building systems that are efficient but unjust, precise but unkind, optimal but hollow.

To move forward, we must reframe optimisation from a pursuit of perfect outcomes to a commitment to meaningful process. That process must be inclusive, transparent, and grounded in moral pluralism. It must recognise that efficiency is not inherently ethical, and that longevity without dignity is not a victory. It must make space for stories, for exceptions, for disagreement, for change.

Ultimately, the question "Who decides what matters?" is not a threat to progress. It is its compass. Without it, we navigate by metrics that glow but do not guide. With it, we chart a future of AI in healthcare that serves not only the system, but the soul of care itself.

Letting Go of the God View

One of the quietest but most consequential shifts in the evolution of healthcare is the rising expectation that uncertainty is a flaw to be engineered away. Decision-support systems powered by artificial intelligence are designed to clarify, accelerate, and optimise choices. Their promise is not simply greater efficiency, but epistemic authority—a clinical clarity immune to bias, fatigue, or oversight. Yet in the attempt to mechanise wisdom, we risk displacing something more fundamental: humility.

Medicine has never been an exact science. It is a field defined as much by probability as by principle. At its best, it acknowledges the plural logics of biology, psyche, social context, and time. Yet, the current wave of computational systems has ushered in a new epistemology—one that privileges predictability, pattern recognition, and probabilistic control. The result is a creeping aspiration toward omniscience: the *God view*—a system's-eye perspective that promises to see more, know better, and decide faster than any single human can.

This epistemic arrogance is not unique to healthcare. It permeates the broader field of AI, where God's-eye metaphors—omniscient databases, total surveillance, predictive policing—are marketed not as dystopias but as solutions. Yet in medicine, the stakes are more intimate. When a machine claims to know what is best for your body, your mind, your life, its conclusions carry not just technical weight but moral gravity. Patients and clinicians alike are increasingly being asked to defer not to shared judgment, but to algorithmic certainty.

And yet that certainty is often illusory. The most advanced diagnostic models still depend on training data riddled with gaps, biases, and historical inequities. Prognostic tools are frequently blind to psychosocial variables that resist quantification—grief, resilience, social connection, spiritual meaning. Clinical datasets privilege what is measurable over what is meaningful, formalised over felt. A system may identify a 78% chance of surgical success, but it cannot compute the emotional cost of recovery in a patient who lives alone, or the ethical discomfort of an intervention that prolongs life but diminishes dignity.

Moreover, complexity is not just a limitation of our models—it is an ontological fact. Human health is not a closed system. It is porous, dynamic, situated in time and culture. The interplay of genetic predisposition, environmental exposure, behavioural habit, economic constraint, and interpersonal care cannot be fully disaggregated, much less rendered tractable by code. The idea that more data will simply resolve ambiguity mistakes the quantity of information for the quality of insight.

Letting go of the God view, then, is not about rejecting technology. It is about resisting its seduction as an oracle. It is an invitation to design systems that support rather than supplant human discernment. Systems that acknowledge doubt, accommodate dissent, and make space for dialogue. Systems that treat uncertainty not as error but as signal—evidence that we are engaging with the real, the particular, the alive.

One promising avenue is the design of *explainable AI* not merely to justify outputs, but to expose reasoning pathways in ways that allow clinicians to contest, revise, or contextualise them. This shifts the frame from answer provision to collaborative interpretation. Another is the integration of *soft data*—patient narratives, clinician notes, family observations—into models that traditionally prioritise numeric abstraction. Such approaches reassert the value of the qualitative, the anecdotal, the emotionally charged. They do not eliminate ambiguity, but they make it legible.

There is also a critical role for institutional humility. Health systems that embrace the provisional rather than the prescriptive create space for learning, for revision, for saying "we don't know yet." Consider the COVID-19 pandemic, where rapid modelling tools provided invaluable forecasts—but also revealed how fragile those forecasts became in the face of emergent variants, human behaviour, and political response. In countries where public health communication acknowledged the limits of certainty and updated guidance transparently, public trust was more likely to be preserved.

Contrast this with settings where AI systems have been deployed as triage gatekeepers. In one case study from the UK, a predictive tool designed to optimise emergency room allocation deprioritised patients with certain disabilities based on past hospital utilisation, assuming a lower potential benefit from aggressive intervention. The system was statistically sound, but ethically questionable. It failed to accommodate the lived complexity of those patients' conditions. More crucially, it displaced the clinician's discretion—their capacity to weigh, question, and push back.

To support rather than override uncertainty requires rethinking how we structure accountability. We must move away from a model where AI systems function as clinical arbiters, to one where they serve as epistemic companions—offering insight, not instruction. This may mean deliberately slowing down certain decision processes, allowing time for reflection, second opinions, or patient discussion. It may mean building interfaces that highlight confidence intervals, disagreements between models, or areas where data is sparse or contested. It certainly means retraining clinicians not simply to trust or distrust AI, but to engage with it critically, as they would a human colleague with a different specialty or worldview.

There are deeper cultural shifts to be made as well. We must decouple technological sophistication from moral superiority. Just because a system is advanced does not mean it is appropriate. Just because it is consistent does not mean it is fair. Just because it reduces variation does not mean it respects life's nuance. The fetishisation of optimisation often hides a flattening of care—a redefinition of good medicine as reproducible rather than responsive.

None of this implies abandoning AI in healthcare. Rather, it is a call to maturity. We do not need systems that pretend to know everything. We need systems that help us ask better questions. We need tools that widen the aperture of judgment, that illuminate what is known and what is unknowable, and that leave room for the moral, emotional, and situational reasoning that defines care at its best.

Humility, in this context, is not weakness. It is epistemic integrity. It acknowledges that even the most powerful models cannot eliminate uncertainty without eliminating humanity. It reminds us that precision is not the same as wisdom, and that clarity is not the same as compassion. Most of all, it affirms the central truth that health, unlike code, is not something to be solved, but to be lived with—tended to, interpreted, and sometimes endured.

Letting go of the God view does not mean surrendering rigour or abandoning hope. It means recognising that real strength lies not in knowing everything, but in knowing where to stop, where to listen, and where to say: here is what we see—and here is what we still don't understand. That shared space of uncertainty is not a failure. It is the ground of trust. And in that space, human care can do what no system ever fully will.

Chapter 10
Reclaiming the Human in Care

It is entirely possible to meet every measurable target in modern healthcare and yet leave the patient feeling unseen. Systems may run smoothly, diagnoses may be precise, algorithms optimised—but the person at the centre can still feel overlooked, misread, or unheard. This is not a failure of technology alone; it reflects a deeper tension between technical sophistication and ethical imagination. As machine learning reshapes hospitals and clinics, a quiet countercurrent emerges, one that insists humans cannot be reduced to data points—that story, meaning, and relationship must remain central. This chapter dives into that current with both urgency and care.

At its core lies a deceptively simple premise: care is not merely what we do for patients; it is how we come to understand them. And understanding requires more than numbers. It demands narrative, attentiveness, and the willingness to encounter what cannot be quantified. The human presence in care is not a nostalgic relic; it is the very condition of medicine's moral legitimacy. Without it, we are managing processes, not practising care.

AI has brought remarkable gains—risk prediction, automated triage, diagnostic modelling—but it also carries a quiet erosion. These systems standardise inputs and outputs according to assumptions often left implicit. They excel at what can be measured, yet too often ignore what matters most: the texture of suffering, the meaning of illness, the patient's history, culture, dignity, and aspirations. Personalisation driven solely by biometric data or preference algorithms risks becoming a hollow proxy for personhood. A treatment path optimised statistically may overlook what the patient values most—time at home, spiritual reconciliation, or simply the chance to say farewell. Technology, well-intentioned, can thus be structurally indifferent.

This is not a call for nostalgia, but for reinvention. Around the globe, clinicians, designers, and researchers are asking: what if narrative were treated as signal, not noise? From embedding patient stories in electronic records to training AI on ethnographic community data, these efforts rescue innovation from reductionism. When a patient's voice enters the digital record—not as a checkbox or sentiment score, but as a living account of goals and context—clinical decisions gain nuance, empathy, and moral grounding. Compliance becomes collaboration.

For clinicians, this shift is profound. In a world where machines sort, rank, and predict with uncanny accuracy, the human practitioner's role becomes interpretive. Beyond relaying results or following protocols, the modern clinician must act as translator—mediating between algorithmic logic and embodied experience. This requires capacities no dataset can teach: emotional literacy, cultural sensitivity, and the courage to hold uncertainty without defaulting to control. Consultation becomes conversation, not interrogation.

Sceptics may claim such ideals are impractical in strained systems. Yet the emerging field of technologies of listening challenges that notion. Ambient voice tools now reduce documentation burdens, freeing clinicians to give undivided attention. Participatory platforms allow patients to co-design their care plans. Wearables detect subtle behavioural shifts, signalling distress or early relapse. The aim is not to humanise machines, but to de-mechanise care.

The urgency is greatest at life's margins. In end-of-life contexts, metrics like survival or readmission often conflict with what patients truly need: presence, attention, and acknowledgment. Here, the most sophisticated system is one that creates space for silence, for story, for reflection. The care that matters is not the fastest, but the one that grasps the human condition.

Even in early diagnosis, reductionism can dominate. AI may detect a tumour before symptoms arise—but detection alone is insufficient. Decisions about treatment intensity, lifestyle changes, or surveillance require human judgement. Clinicians must engage fully, not as command-and-control authorities, but as partners guiding patients through uncertainty. The future is not automation in lieu of judgment; it is co-creation.

This chapter unfolds across four intertwined themes. First, it examines embedding narrative into digital infrastructure, showing how structured stories can travel alongside data to inform decisions with context and ethical depth. Second, it reimagines clinicians as interpreters of meaning, cultivating literacies in uncertainty, culture, and relational nuance. Third, it explores technologies of listening—tools that allow presence, co-reflection, and attentiveness to flourish within clinical workflows. Finally, it critiques prevailing personalisation paradigms, arguing that individualisation is not equivalent to understanding; personhood-centred care places values, relationships, and autonomy at its core.

To reclaim the human in care is not to reject technology, but to guide it toward maturity. Intelligence does not equal wisdom, and tools that touch lives must be shaped not only by capability, but by ethical intention. The question is not whether machines will become more human—it is whether humans will remain central to what care truly means.

In the chapters ahead, readers will encounter both the urgency and possibility of this reclamation. This is not sentimentalism; it is a call to design, train, govern, and imagine healthcare in ways that honour the full depth of human need.

If the future of medicine is to be intelligent, it must also be profoundly, deliberately human.

Reintroducing Narrative into the System

In a hospital ward in Denmark, a young woman diagnosed with multiple sclerosis tells her physician that her priority is not controlling the next lesion or extending her prognosis—it's being well enough to read to her children every night. The neurologist nods, prescribes a new medication, and updates the electronic health record. But the patient's words—her story, her purpose—go undocumented, unanalysed, unvalued by the very system meant to support her. She leaves with a care plan tailored to her biomarkers but not to her meaning. And yet it is that unrecorded fragment—the bedtime story—that defines the success or failure of her care.

This is not an edge case. It is the norm. Clinical information systems, particularly those governed by AI and predictive analytics, have been designed for efficiency, interoperability, and standardisation. These are important aims. But what they have displaced is equally important: narrative context, patient voice, cultural texture, and the lived logic of illness. *The absence of patient story in healthcare data is not a technical oversight—it is a systemic erasure.* Reintroducing narrative into these systems is not about sentiment; it is about restoring medicine's epistemic balance.

The medical record, once a narrative artefact handwritten by physicians to capture the trajectory of a patient's illness, has been transformed into a structured data matrix. Checkboxes, dropdowns, numeric fields. The format is optimised for billing, for epidemiological tracking, for clinical trials. It is not optimised for human understanding. The result is a record that contains what is easily measurable but often omits what is meaningfully human. Patients appear as problems to be solved, not people to be understood.

The integration of artificial intelligence into health systems has only deepened this reduction. Predictive algorithms rely on structured, sanitised inputs. Natural language processing systems still struggle to parse the subtlety of narrative nuance—humour, irony, cultural idioms, metaphor. And so these data are filtered out, deemed irrelevant or unreliable. But this absence has consequences. When an algorithm recommends aggressive intervention based on disease progression alone, without consideration of a patient's aversion to hospitalisation or desire for home-based palliative care, the care becomes misaligned with the person. *Precision without meaning is precision misplaced.*

Yet a growing number of initiatives are resisting this trend. In the Netherlands, the "Mijn Verhaal" pilot project allows patients to record short narratives about their lives, goals, and fears, which are then embedded into their digital health records. These narratives are not summarised or reinterpreted by clinicians—they are included in the patient's own voice. When a new specialist accesses the file, they begin with story, not symptom. Early evaluations suggest this improves trust, enhances shared decision-making, and even reduces unnecessary tests. The story functions not as decoration but as data—data of a different epistemology.

In the United States, researchers at Stanford are building models that combine clinical data with patient-authored illness narratives to train machine learning systems in values-aligned decision support. Instead of optimising for longevity alone, these models are being tested to align with preferences such as functional independence, spiritual peace, or family time. This shift requires not only technological redesign but *ethical reorientation*: a recognition that optimisation, to be meaningful, must reflect the person's own vision of the good.

The implications extend beyond technology. Medical training, too, is undergoing re-evaluation. At institutions such as McGill and King's College London, narrative medicine is being integrated into curricula—not as a soft skill, but as a clinical tool. Students are taught to read literature, write reflective narratives, and conduct "narrative interviews" with patients. These exercises are not intended to displace science, but to *expand its scope*, equipping future clinicians to interpret suffering as more than a checklist of complaints.

Critics sometimes argue that narrative is too subjective, too idiosyncratic, too difficult to scale. But this objection misreads the purpose of story. Narrative is not a replacement for data—it is a necessary companion. A story offers texture to the trajectory of illness, reveals the meanings people attach to their symptoms, and situates clinical decisions within the contours of a life. A cancer diagnosis may mean statistical risk to a model, but to the patient it may mean the loss of a future imagined, of unfinished conversations, of children not yet grown. *To ignore this is to mistake medicine for mechanics.*

Indeed, the cultural implications are significant. In Indigenous communities across Australia and Canada, story is not a communication method—it is a knowledge system. It encodes history, ethics, cosmology. When healthcare systems engage with these communities using purely clinical or statistical frameworks, they not only miss the patient's context—they risk replicating colonial logics of erasure. Some projects, like the "Two-Eyed Seeing" framework in Nova Scotia, attempt to hold both Western clinical models and Indigenous ways of knowing together. In these settings, narrative is not a supplement to care; it is *care itself.*

Designing systems that support this integration is complex but not impossible. It requires shifts in interface design, data architecture, and regulatory frameworks. Instead of asking, "What symptoms brought you here today?" electronic intake systems might begin with, "What do we need to understand about your life to help you best?" Instead of structuring data solely by diagnosis and treatment, systems might create parallel tracks for values, fears, and goals. These could be as simple as tagged audio clips or as structured as modular narrative fields. What matters is not format but *epistemic legitimacy*—whether the system treats this information as central or peripheral.

There are risks to navigate. When patient narratives become data, they may be mined, misinterpreted, or even weaponised by insurers or automated systems. Safeguards must be robust. Consent must be explicit. Interpretation must be human-guided. But these challenges are not arguments against narrative—they are arguments for doing it responsibly. *The solution to bad use of story is not less story; it is deeper care in how stories are held.*

The philosophical core of this shift is the belief that health is not only about what the body endures, but how the person makes sense of that endurance. Illness disrupts not just cells, but meaning. And healing, at its best, is a collaborative reconstruction of that meaning—between patient, clinician, and sometimes machine. This reconstruction is impossible without story. A system that cannot hear patients is a system that cannot heal them fully.

As AI continues to transform the clinical landscape, we face a choice. We can build systems that amplify existing reductionisms, training them to do more of what we already do—faster, cheaper, narrower. Or we can use this moment to recalibrate, to design technologies that honour complexity and support the interpretive work of care. The reintroduction of narrative is not a sentimental gesture—it is a structural correction. It is an insistence that care must begin with listening, and that *what matters to the patient must matter to the system.*

The road ahead is not straightforward. Embedding narrative into health IT infrastructures will require innovation, funding, policy reform, and sustained cultural change. But the direction is clear. We are moving not just toward more intelligent systems, but toward more *humane* ones. Systems that do not simply process inputs, but attend to lives. That do not merely personalise, but *understand*. And in doing so, make room for a kind of medicine that is not only smart, but wise.

The New Role of the Clinician as Interpreter

When a patient receives a treatment recommendation from an AI-powered system—one that confidently ranks therapeutic options based on survival rates, genetic compatibility, and cost efficiency—they are not just receiving a clinical suggestion. They are being handed an outcome calculated in silence, absent of context, values, or lived complexity. It is here, in the margin between algorithmic certainty and human ambiguity, that the clinician now stands—not solely as diagnostician, nor merely as technician, but as *interpreter*. In this evolving role, the clinician translates machine logic into human meaning, and patient narrative into actionable care. It is a role that is not auxiliary to medicine—it is its epistemological centre.

The notion that AI could outperform clinicians in diagnostic accuracy was once provocative; today it is increasingly accepted in specific domains. From radiology to dermatology to pathology, machine learning systems have shown remarkable proficiency in pattern recognition. Yet the idea that AI could *replace* clinicians is a misreading of both technology's capabilities and medicine's purpose. *Diagnosis is not understanding*. Prediction is not interpretation. And care is not computation. What patients require—what they have always required—is someone who can help them make sense of what is happening to their bodies and their lives, in language that acknowledges both science and story.

This interpretive function cannot be automated. It demands skills that are deeply human and profoundly contextual: listening, reframing, contextualising, negotiating uncertainty. A machine may predict that a particular chemotherapy regimen offers a 12% increase in five-year survival. But it cannot assess whether that outcome is meaningful to a 76-year-old patient who values time at home with grandchildren more than time spent in a treatment ward. Nor can it weigh the existential cost of side effects that erode identity. The clinician, in conversation with the patient, must hold both sets of knowledge—clinical data and personal values—and *mediate between them*.

Interpretation, in this context, is not a soft skill—it is the core clinical act. It involves understanding that health is not a universal equation but a personal calculus. It involves articulating risks not only numerically but narratively, helping patients situate statistical projections within the contours of their lives. This demands fluency in medical epistemology and in human conversation; the ability to read a chart and to read a room.

In practice, this role manifests in myriad ways. In palliative care, where treatment decisions often defy the logic of optimisation, clinicians routinely reframe questions away from "What's the best intervention?" to "What matters most to you now?" In genetic counselling, where AI systems can identify pathogenic variants with astonishing speed, the challenge is not detection but discussion—guiding families through uncertain probabilities and life-altering choices. And in primary care, where patients often present with symptoms that resist clear categorisation, the clinician must interpret not only data but distress, translating discomfort into diagnosis, and diagnosis into a shared plan.

To support this interpretive function, healthcare systems must shift their incentives and architectures. Time, the clinician's most valuable interpretive tool, is currently the most constrained. Decision-support tools, if poorly integrated, can overwhelm rather than assist. Many clinicians describe feeling trapped between the velocity of automated recommendations and the slowness required for real conversation. Systems must be designed not to expedite decisions, but to *deepen deliberation*. That means user interfaces that surface not just outputs but rationales. It means alerts that invite questions, not just clicks. And it means workflows that preserve space for dialogue.

Training must evolve in parallel. Medical education has historically privileged the accumulation of knowledge over its contextual application. In an AI-augmented future, knowledge will be abundant. What will differentiate excellent clinicians is their interpretive capacity: their ability to discern when an algorithm's recommendation aligns with a patient's life, and when it does not. Curricula must therefore prioritise critical thinking, ethical reasoning, communication theory, and narrative competence. These are not "add-ons" to the scientific core—they are its indispensable counterpart in the clinic of tomorrow.

Some argue that interpretation introduces unacceptable subjectivity into an already complex system. But this concern misunderstands the nature of medicine. Clinical decisions are never purely objective; they are always situated. Evidence-based guidelines are necessary but not sufficient. They must be interpreted in light of patient preference, comorbidity, socioeconomic context, and cultural meaning. An AI system may suggest anticoagulation for atrial fibrillation based on guidelines, but a clinician must interpret whether that recommendation makes sense for a patient with high fall risk, or for someone who cannot afford the prescription.

Moreover, interpretive medicine is not antithetical to rigour. On the contrary, it demands a more expansive rigour—one that integrates empirical evidence with existential insight. It requires clinicians to be as skilled at discerning patterns in people as they are at interpreting patterns in data. It calls for intellectual humility: the recognition that the same set of facts can yield different decisions when viewed through different human lenses.

There are powerful precedents for this model. In the humanities, the role of the interpreter is well established. A literary critic does not merely summarise a text—they unpack its tensions, trace its themes, explore its ambiguities. Similarly, a clinician-as-interpreter navigates the space between biomedical input and patient response, holding space for paradox, ambivalence, and evolving understanding. In this view, *care is not merely administered—it is co-constructed.*

This shift is not only epistemological but ethical. When clinicians abdicate the interpretive role—whether due to time pressure, over-reliance on algorithms, or institutional inertia—patients are left to navigate meaning alone. This can result in care that is technically excellent but emotionally alienating. It can result in consent that is legally sufficient but morally thin. And it can erode trust, not because of error, but because of the absence of empathy. Interpretation restores that trust. It says: I see your data, but more importantly, I see *you.*

The rise of AI in healthcare is not a threat to this role—it is an invitation to refine it. As machines assume more of the cognitive load, clinicians are freed to focus on the interpretive, relational, and ethical dimensions of care. This is not a diminishment of medical authority—it is its deepening. It acknowledges that what patients seek is not only accuracy, but *understanding*; not only prediction, but partnership.

The future of medicine will not be a contest between human and machine, but a collaboration. In this collaboration, clinicians will not compete with AI on speed or memory—they will complement it with meaning. They will serve as interpreters of both data and desire, mediating between the logics of computation and the logics of care. And in doing so, they will reclaim the heart of medicine—not as a technical domain alone, but as a deeply human practice grounded in presence, purpose, and translation.

As we design the next generation of clinical systems, this vision must guide us. We must build tools that illuminate patterns *without obscuring persons*. We must resist the seduction of frictionless automation when friction is where discernment lives. And we must invest not only in faster algorithms, but in more thoughtful clinicians—equipped, empowered, and trusted to interpret, always, with wisdom and care.

Technologies of Listening

A diagnostic decision may be shaped by lab results, imaging, and predictive models, but trust is shaped by something less quantifiable: whether the patient feels heard. Despite the exponential rise of data-driven medicine, healthcare remains a fundamentally relational practice. And yet, much of modern health technology is still designed for extraction—capturing, categorising, and computing patient information—while overlooking the deeper human act of *listening*. The next frontier in care is not only about developing smarter algorithms, but about cultivating *technologies of attention*—tools and practices that elevate presence, deepen empathy, and prioritise meaningful conversation over mechanistic throughput. To listen well is not to passively receive; it is to actively honour what matters to another. In healthcare, that act is both clinical and moral.

Consider a typical electronic health record (EHR) interface. Its design prioritises coding efficiency, billing compliance, and biomedical detail, yet rarely encourages the nuanced capture of patient values, fears, or personal context. A 58-year-old woman with heart failure may appear as an amalgam of vital signs, medication lists, and procedural histories. Her desire to stay mobile enough to dance at her daughter's wedding is likely nowhere to be found. Her story exists, but the system has no field for it. This absence is not neutral—it shapes what care is possible.

True listening in healthcare must be *designed for*, not assumed. That requires shifting from systems optimised for throughput to systems attuned to meaning. It demands interfaces that capture not just symptoms, but stories; not just choices, but the reasoning behind them. Some emerging technologies are beginning to move in this direction—notably natural language processing tools that can summarise clinician-patient conversations to preserve nuance without flattening meaning, or voice-recording systems that document tone, pauses, and emotional cues alongside content. But the challenge is not merely technical; it is conceptual. *What counts as data?* What deserves to be captured? And how might we design for presence, not just precision?

The answer may lie in reframing "listening" as an act of *clinical intelligence*. A physician who notices that a patient's voice quivers when discussing a treatment option is engaging in data collection—just not the kind traditionally valorised by clinical software. This interpretive listening is essential for surfacing ambivalence, identifying trauma, or uncovering underlying values that might otherwise remain hidden. Some health systems are now experimenting with "narrative summaries" within EHRs—spaces where clinicians or patients themselves can record a guiding story that frames medical data in human terms. In paediatrics, for instance, a mother's note about her son's anxiety around needles may guide the choice of blood draw technique more effectively than any standardised prompt.

Technology can support this kind of attentiveness—but only if built to do so. One example is "OpenNotes," a movement that grants patients access to their clinicians' visit notes. Studies show that when patients read their records, they feel more engaged, spot errors, and often gain new clarity about their care plans. But the practice also nudges clinicians toward greater thoughtfulness in how they document: if the patient will read the note, its tone and language must reflect dignity, clarity, and respect. Listening, in this sense, becomes not only a clinical act but a co-authored one—each note a trace of mutual recognition.

Other innovations embed listening into care workflows more directly. AI-enabled conversation tools like Abridge and Augmedix aim to relieve clinicians of the burden of note-taking during appointments, allowing them to focus fully on the patient. These tools transcribe and summarise visits in real time, freeing cognitive bandwidth for human connection. Early evaluations suggest that when clinicians are not preoccupied with typing, their questions become more exploratory, their tone warmer, their responsiveness sharper. In short, *the presence of listening increases when the technology listens, too.*

Still, these developments raise important ethical and epistemological questions. Who gets to listen? What is listened for? And whose voice is privileged when stories conflict? Consider language interpretation services—technologically enabled yet frequently underfunded. In the absence of trained interpreters, clinicians often rely on family members or even AI-powered translation apps. But literal translation is not listening; it's transcription. The meaning behind a phrase—its emotional weight, cultural context, and implicit expectations—can be lost without attuned human mediation. Thus, a "technology of listening" must include the infrastructure to support multilingual, multicultural, and cross-contextual understanding. Anything less risks reproducing the asymmetries it seeks to repair.

Equally urgent is the need to listen across time. A patient's story is rarely a single event—it is episodic, evolving, sometimes contradictory. Traditional clinical documentation fragments this narrative into discrete encounters. But new longitudinal tools aim to preserve continuity: digital platforms that track care goals over time, annotate decisions with contextual notes, and highlight shifts in patient values. These systems do not just capture what was said, but *how understanding changed.* They create a record of listening as a dynamic, iterative process.

The importance of this becomes acute in complex or chronic illness, where decisions rarely hinge on a single test result. A person with advanced cancer navigating palliative options may change their mind multiple times. A technology that only logs the final decision misses the terrain traversed—the doubts voiced, the reassurances given, the redefinition of hope. Listening, here, is not a checkbox; it is the architecture of trust.

Even in mental health, where listening is core to therapeutic practice, technology often veers toward surveillance rather than support. Mood-tracking apps, biometric wearables, and behaviour-monitoring tools promise early detection of distress—but they often fail to contextualise experience. A drop in sleep hours may flag risk, but it cannot explain grief. A spike in heart rate may indicate anxiety, or simply a spirited conversation. Designing mental health technologies that listen well means allowing users to annotate their own data, offer subjective framing, and reject reductive interpretations. It means designing not for compliance, but for co-interpretation.

This principle also extends to marginalised communities, who have long experienced medical listening as conditional or extractive. Community health projects that deploy story circles, peer-led data collection, or participatory design models show how technologies of listening can emerge from below—not imposed from above. The HIVE Project in San Francisco, serving women and trans people living with HIV, includes patient narratives as a core part of both clinical records and research protocols. These narratives are not decorative—they guide care. Similarly, Indigenous health programmes in Canada and Australia are using digital storytelling to preserve traditional health knowledge alongside biomedical data. These tools do not just listen to individuals—they listen to cultures.

None of this is a rejection of data science. It is a call to expand our notion of what counts as data, and to design technologies that listen *as clinicians do*: attentively, responsively, ethically. Listening is not a metaphor—it is a skill, a practice, and increasingly, a design requirement.

To build technologies of listening is to acknowledge that care does not begin with treatment. It begins with attention. It begins with the patient who says, "I'm not sure how to explain this," and the clinician who responds, "Take your time." It begins with a system that values that exchange as much as any scan or score. And it continues in the tools that document, amplify, and carry those moments forward—so that the next clinician does not just inherit a chart, but a conversation.

In a healthcare landscape increasingly defined by automation, scaling, and efficiency metrics, the insistence on listening may seem quaint. But it is, in fact, a radical design principle. It asks not only what the system knows, but *how it knows*. It demands technologies that do not just *collect*, but *connect*. And it reorients the purpose of innovation—from answering questions quickly, to understanding people deeply. That is not a luxury. It is the foundation of humane care.

From Personalised to Personhood-Centred Care

Personalisation has become a defining mantra in modern medicine. From genomic tailoring of treatments to AI-powered health recommendations, we are repeatedly told that the future lies in "customised" care—data-driven, targeted, precise. Yet this framing subtly distorts what it means to care. When personalisation is equated solely with predictive accuracy or algorithmic alignment, it risks reducing patients to a set of optimised variables—while eroding the very qualities that make healthcare human. The deeper question, often unasked, is this: personalised *to what end*? To prolong life at any cost? To meet statistical thresholds? To increase system efficiency? Or to serve the lived dignity, values, and agency of the individual?

To move from personalised to *personhood-centred* care is not to reject data or innovation. It is to ground their use in *relationship*, *recognition*, and *shared decision-making*. It is to acknowledge that while a person's genome may inform drug response, it says nothing about what that person hopes for, fears, or finds meaningful. A truly humane health system must do more than predict preferences—it must honour them.

The distinction is not semantic—it is structural. In current practice, personalisation is often achieved by mining historical data to forecast likely choices or outcomes. A diabetic patient may be nudged toward a specific insulin regimen based on biometric patterns. A cancer patient may receive an AI-curated treatment plan optimised for survival probabilities. These interventions may be clinically sound—but if they proceed without dialogue, without co-interpretation, they risk collapsing care into computation. *They confuse tailoring with listening.*

Consider the case of Maria, a 67-year-old woman diagnosed with early-stage breast cancer. Her oncologist presents her with a treatment plan recommended by an algorithm trained on thousands of similar cases. Statistically, it is sound. But Maria hesitates. Her daughter lives abroad, and intensive chemotherapy would make travel difficult. She wonders if a less aggressive treatment, though slightly less effective, might allow her to attend her granddaughter's graduation. The system does not account for this. It was trained on outcomes measured in months of survival, not *moments of meaning*. The algorithm optimises, but it does not understand what matters most.

Maria's story is not rare. It reflects a widespread tension between population-level optimisation and individual-centred values. AI systems are extraordinarily good at

you hope to preserve?" The former is a mirror; the latter is a conversation. The former optimises; the latter honours.

That difference matters most when patients are most vulnerable—when facing uncertainty, contradiction, or loss. Personhood-centred care does not aim to resolve such moments through certainty, but to *accompany them with clarity*. It sees the role of the clinician not just as a fixer, but as a *witness*—to the patient's story, fears, contradictions, and hopes. It measures success not only in outcomes, but in whether the patient felt respected, seen, and involved. Such care may be less tidy, but it is more truthful.

Culturally, this shift has implications beyond the clinic. A personhood-centred system invites healthcare institutions to consider equity not merely in terms of access, but in terms of *dignity*. Marginalised patients—those with disabilities, those from historically excluded groups, those who speak differently or navigate systems with distrust—are often excluded from the personalisation revolution precisely because their data does not fit prevailing models. A rehumanised vision would ask not only how we tailor care, but *whose stories the system is able to hear*.

To be personhood-centred is thus to be pluralistic: to acknowledge that care cannot be standardised because people are not standard. It means designing for *difference*, not deviation—for multiple ways of being well, not one universal algorithm of health. It means returning to a truth long known in practice but often absent in policy: that care is not delivered; it is *co-created*.

This is not a nostalgic appeal to pre-technological medicine. It is a forward-looking demand for *relational intelligence*—a way of building systems that remember what they are for. Personalisation, stripped of personhood, is clever but cold. When rooted in relationship, dignity, and shared meaning, it becomes not just more humane, but more *clinically wise*. And it becomes a reminder that even in the age of precision, the deepest truths in care are still spoken, not calculated.

Chapter 11
Designing the Future We Want

No system arises spontaneously. The trajectory of healthcare will be shaped not only by the sophistication of algorithms, but by the ethical scaffolding that underpins them, the clarity of the values they encode, and the resolve of those who craft them. As artificial intelligence increasingly participates in clinical decisions, operational processes, and patient experiences, the pressing question is no longer whether these tools will be used, but how, why, and for whose benefit. This chapter engages that question directly, advocating a seemingly radical principle: care must be designed, not merely delivered, with human dignity as its foundation and ethical foresight as its compass.

In the rush of innovation, it is tempting to equate capability with desirability. That an AI system can forecast hospital readmissions or generate patient summaries in moments does not in itself validate its justice, transparency, or alignment with patient priorities. Rapid development, alluring though it is, can mask deeper structural hazards: unexamined biases, unintended harms, and the stealthy expansion of dehumanisation in the guise of efficiency. The dialogue must mature beyond admiration for technical prowess, moving toward a deliberate examination of purpose.

Ethical integration cannot be relegated to post-deployment audits or isolated technical adjustments. It begins at the design table, as a multidimensional practice drawing on philosophy, sociology, clinical insight, and lived experience. This chapter frames a working triad—accountability, explainability, and human alignment—as criteria that must be embedded throughout AI development, deployment, and governance.

Accountability demands that algorithmic outcomes be traceable to human judgement, morally as well as technically. Who bears responsibility when harm occurs? Who has authority to challenge, override, or suspend a model? Systems without robust accountability do more than invite error; they erode trust, disempowering users from clinicians to patients. Explainability requires that AI systems be intelligible not just to programmers, but to those affected by their recommendations. A black-box model, however accurate, should not dictate life-altering decisions without mechanisms for scrutiny, dialogue, or dissent. Human alignment questions whether a system's objectives—whether efficiency, cost reduction, or throughput—cohere with the intricate, often conflicting values of human well-being. Optimisation, in this light, is never neutral; it is inherently ethical.

Yet AI does not exist in a vacuum—it operates within institutions. To advance genuinely person-centred care, healthcare organisations must resist the temptation to automate at the expense of conversation. They must recognise that metrics, though powerful, are imperfect proxies for meaning. What is measured often dictates what is prioritised, irrespective of ethical import. Institutions that cultivate compassion must monitor not only algorithmic drift, but mission drift: the gradual displacement of relational care by throughput, documentation, and compliance. Culture, in this sense, is the infrastructure beneath the infrastructure. If AI is to reflect humility, empathy, and pluralism, institutional policies, educational curricula, and funding priorities must reinforce these values at every level.

This responsibility is not the sole province of technologists. The stakes are too high. Patients, clinicians, ethicists, regulators, and communities all have roles in shaping the design language of care. Yet most are handed tools, not criteria; outputs, not questions. A central aim of this chapter is to provide practical agency: a toolkit for those at any point in the system to ask the right questions, challenge assumptions, and advocate for humane design. Which values underpin this model? What trade-offs informed its construction? Who stands to benefit—and who may be marginalised? How can coercive digital nudges be resisted, vendor claims evaluated, and systemic change advocated? Democratising healthcare technology begins with demystification.

Importantly, this chapter is not merely defensive. It does not dwell solely on preventing harm, but on cultivating possibility. Imagine AI systems that do not imitate care but enrich it. Conversational agents trained not merely on medical texts but on authentic patient narratives, supporting rather than supplanting human dialogue. Predictive tools deployed to expand choice rather than constrict it, to illuminate uncertainty rather than conceal it. Success measured not solely in throughput or cost, but in patient dignity, comprehension, clinician trust, and equitable access.

The future we desire will not arrive unbidden. It must be articulated, contested, and deliberately constructed. And it begins with clarity. Recognition that technology is never neutral—it amplifies what is rewarded, overlooked, or feared. Discipline to ask not just what works, but what matters. Humility to acknowledge that care is a human art, one no system, however intelligent, can replace. Presence, moral attention, and interpretive engagement remain irreplaceable.

This chapter serves, at heart, as a manifesto for deliberate design. Healthcare's digital architecture is being drafted now, often invisibly, by those far removed from clinic floors or patient bedsides. But it need not remain so. Readers are participants in this process. Whether selecting tools as practitioners, shaping policy as regulators, or advocating for humane treatment as patients, each of us carries a portion of the future in our hands. The task ahead is not merely to anticipate change—but to shape it intentionally, wisely, and with care.

A Framework for Ethical Integration

It is no longer sufficient to ask whether a healthcare algorithm works; we must now ask *for whom* it works, *on what terms*, and *at what cost to human dignity*. As artificial intelligence continues its expansion into diagnostic tools, clinical decision support, resource triage, and even conversational interfaces, its promises of speed and accuracy are too often accepted as synonymous with progress. But technical prowess without ethical scrutiny risks amplifying harm under the guise of help. The future of AI in healthcare will be shaped not merely by breakthroughs in data science but by the principles we embed in its design—principles that govern who benefits, who is left behind, and how we define good care. This is the work of ethical integration, and it demands more than vague commitments to "doing no harm." It calls for rigor, transparency, and an unwavering alignment with human values.

One of the central challenges in evaluating AI tools is the seductive neutrality of metrics. Optimising for efficiency or predictive accuracy may seem inherently valuable, but these metrics often conceal contested assumptions about what healthcare is for. A system that minimises hospital admissions, for instance, may be framed as cost-effective—but it may also result in fewer interventions for vulnerable patients who lack access to preventative care. A triage algorithm that "rationalises" emergency room traffic may inadvertently downgrade patients with complex symptoms that do not match its training data. The point is not to discard optimisation but to interrogate it: *what is being optimised, and who gets to decide?* Without ethical scaffolding, even well-intentioned AI systems can drift into forms of structural bias, epistemic injustice, or techno-determinism.

Three pillars—*accountability, explainability,* and *human alignment*—form the backbone of a robust framework for ethical integration. Each pillar acts as a necessary constraint on what AI can be permitted to do in environments where stakes are irreducibly human.

Accountability is the condition under which any system must operate if it is to be ethically and democratically legitimate. In healthcare, accountability must extend beyond the engineers who build algorithms to the institutions that deploy them and the professionals who interpret their outputs. This includes traceable audit trails for clinical decisions influenced by AI, formal channels for contestation when harms occur, and governance structures that include patient voices—not merely as "user feedback" but as moral stakeholders. Too often, systems are deployed in grey zones of responsibility, where outcomes are attributed to probabilistic error or insufficient training data, rather than system design. A meaningful framework for accountability must be both retrospective and prospective: it must assess past outcomes, but also proactively constrain AI capabilities in high-risk contexts.

Explainability is not just a technical goal—it is a moral imperative. Patients and clinicians alike must be able to understand the basis of AI recommendations, particularly when they intersect with diagnoses, prognoses, or treatment pathways. Yet many current systems rely on black-box models, where even their developers cannot fully articulate how a given output was reached. This opacity erodes trust and impedes meaningful consent. Efforts toward explainable AI (XAI) have advanced through visualisation tools, rule-based approximations, and post-hoc interpretability techniques, but much of this work remains concentrated in technical silos. What is needed now is a shift toward *relational explainability*—a model where the act of explanation is adapted to the recipient's context, language, and cognitive needs. A good explanation in medicine is not a data dump; it is a narrative that allows a person to make informed choices about their body and future.

Human alignment is perhaps the most ambitious pillar, because it requires AI systems to serve not merely as neutral tools, but as instruments aligned with the values and goals of the people they affect. In medicine, this means more than avoiding harm—it means supporting flourishing. It involves designing systems that accommodate uncertainty, respect patient autonomy, and uphold the dignity of those with non-normative experiences of health and illness. Aligning AI with human values is not a one-time calibration; it is an ongoing process of negotiation, reflection, and responsiveness. This demands interdisciplinary involvement—philosophers, sociologists, disability advocates, clinicians, and patients must all have a seat at the design table. Human alignment also means recognising that values are plural and sometimes in conflict: autonomy may pull against safety; cost-efficiency may compete with comprehensiveness. Ethical integration requires deliberative mechanisms that make these tensions visible and navigable, rather than papered over by default metrics.

A practical example of this tension can be found in the development of predictive models for mental health crises. Some AI systems claim to detect suicidal ideation based on social media activity, biometric data, or electronic health records. But what should be done with such predictions? Should intervention be automatic? Who interprets the data? What are the risks of false positives or unjustified surveillance? These are not just technical design questions; they are deeply ethical ones. Accountability here would demand that decisions made on the basis of such predictions are traceable, contestable, and subject to review. Explainability would require that the individuals affected understand why a particular flag was raised. Human alignment would insist that the system be sensitive to stigma, contextual nuance, and the lived experience of those in psychological distress. Anything less risks turning care into coercion.

Another example comes from the use of AI in radiology. Deep learning models now outperform some specialists in detecting early-stage cancers from imaging data. Impressive, but what happens when the machine finds something a human misses? Does the clinician override their judgement? Does the patient get told of every AI-flagged anomaly, even if it's clinically ambiguous? If AI recommendations become the standard, are doctors liable for not following them? These questions show how ethical integration cannot be retrofitted after deployment. The system's purpose, its scope of authority, and its limits must be designed *from the outset* with accountability, explainability, and human alignment as first principles.

There is a temptation to outsource moral complexity to algorithms under the banner of objectivity. But data is never raw; it is collected, cleaned, and labelled by humans within systems shaped by economic pressures, historical biases, and cultural assumptions. Optimisation targets are rarely neutral. Even something as seemingly uncontroversial as reducing wait times can have unintended effects if it incentivises hospitals to triage low-complexity cases over more urgent but resource-intensive ones. The question is not whether AI should optimise—it is whether we can govern that optimisation wisely. That requires more than technical expertise; it requires moral imagination.

Importantly, ethical integration is not a checklist. It is not satisfied by including a line about "fairness" in a product brief or hiring a part-time ethicist. It is a paradigm shift—one that sees ethical reflection as intrinsic to innovation, not as a compliance burden or PR exercise. Institutions must invest not just in engineers, but in ethical leadership. Medical schools and data science programmes must train professionals to think across disciplinary lines. Regulatory bodies must develop new frameworks that evaluate not just safety and efficacy, but the ethical contours of deployment. And perhaps most critically, patients and the public must be treated not as passive recipients of AI-powered care but as active participants in its design and governance.

As we move deeper into an age of AI-infused healthcare, we face a choice: to accept tools that deliver convenience at the cost of care, or to insist on systems that embody our highest commitments to human dignity, trust, and relational meaning. The latter path is more difficult. It will slow some deployments. It will demand uncomfortable conversations. But it is the only path that deserves to be called progress. *Ethical integration is not an accessory to innovation—it is its conscience.* Without it, the future of care will be fast, clever, and inhumane. With it, we may yet build something worthy of the name "healthcare."

Building Institutions That Resist Dehumanisation

There is a persistent risk in modern healthcare that the very technologies developed to serve human needs will gradually erode the human experience itself. Nowhere is this paradox more evident than in the rapid integration of artificial intelligence and digital tools into health systems. These technologies promise efficiency, consistency, and precision. Yet without intentional design, cultural accountability, and institutional vision, they can produce environments that feel sterile, impersonal, and emotionally indifferent. *To avoid such outcomes, we must focus not merely on designing better tools—but on building institutions capable of resisting dehumanisation at every level.*

Dehumanisation in healthcare rarely begins with malice. It begins with misalignment. It begins when clinicians are pressured to prioritise data input over meaningful conversation. It begins when health systems reward throughput over thoughtfulness, when education trains for compliance rather than critical discernment, and when policy defaults to cost-efficiency at the expense of care. These are not flaws in the algorithms alone—they are systemic choices, embedded in how we structure our institutions, incentivise behaviour, and interpret what it means to be well.

What makes an institution humane is not its technology—but its posture toward the human condition. A hospital can be full of advanced systems and yet be profoundly alienating if it fails to see the patient as more than a case. Conversely, a modest clinic with limited resources can create a deeply human space if it preserves the dignity, autonomy, and complexity of the individuals it serves. The challenge is to ensure that as institutions evolve technologically, they do not regress ethically. That requires deliberate work in three domains: policy, education, and organisational culture.

Policy as Moral Architecture

Policies are not merely bureaucratic scaffolds; they are declarations of values in operational form. They tell us what is permissible, what is rewarded, and what is invisible. For institutions aiming to integrate AI without dehumanising care, policy must function as moral architecture—shaping the behaviour of both machines and people toward accountable, relational, and context-sensitive outcomes.

Consider consent frameworks. In many systems, consent is a formality—a one-time checkbox preceding treatment or data sharing. A humane institution reimagines consent as an ongoing conversation. This shift would require policy that mandates transparency not just at the point of data collection, but throughout the continuum of care. Patients should be informed when AI is influencing clinical decisions, be empowered to ask questions, and have access to clear explanations of how their data is being used. This form of procedural justice does not emerge from software—it emerges from governance.

Moreover, policies must actively resist the path of least resistance. When AI tools default to optimising for efficiency or risk-reduction without examining patient-defined outcomes, the system drifts toward technocratic paternalism. To counteract this, institutional policies should include mechanisms for value-based review—committees or boards that evaluate not just whether a tool *works*, but whether it *serves*. These reviews should include diverse stakeholders, including patients, ethicists, frontline clinicians, and communities most at risk of marginalisation.

Education as Ethical Formation

Education is where the future of care begins—not in devices, but in people. Yet current training often fails to equip health professionals with the interpretive skills required to mediate between technological complexity and human nuance. Too often, clinicians are trained to trust systems more than stories, and to defer to algorithmic outputs without interrogating their assumptions.

A humane institution invests in ethical formation as rigorously as it does in technical proficiency. That means embedding moral reasoning, critical AI literacy, and narrative competence into curricula. Future clinicians must understand not just how to use a clinical decision support tool, but *what it omits*, *how it frames the problem*, and *whose priorities it encodes*. They must be taught to ask: *Whose voice is missing here? What does this output assume about what matters?*

Some pioneering medical schools are already making this shift. Initiatives in narrative medicine, reflective practice, and interdisciplinary ethics are reframing the role of the clinician from diagnostician to dialogical partner. Likewise, data science programmes are beginning to integrate modules on fairness, explainability, and human-centred design. These efforts are critical—but still too rare. If AI is to become a central force in healthcare, then *understanding its limits and social implications must become a core professional competency, not a niche elective.*

Culture as the Soil of Care

Policy and education set the rules and knowledge base of a system—but culture shapes its soul. Organisational culture determines what behaviours are celebrated, what kinds of questions are safe to ask, and whether people feel seen or sorted. It is within culture that the deepest forms of dehumanisation—or rehumanisation—take root.

A culture that resists dehumanisation is one that protects the space for human presence. That means designing work environments where clinicians have time to listen, where patient complexity is not seen as a scheduling burden, and where uncertainty is not punished but respected. It also means cultivating humility at the institutional level—recognising that no metric, however elegant, captures the full experience of illness or healing.

Language is a powerful cultural lever. How institutions talk about patients and technologies influences how people within them behave. When electronic health records refer to patients as "users," or when dashboards reduce well-being to compliance scores, it signals a detachment from the embodied reality of care. Leaders can shift culture by insisting on language that honours personhood, by celebrating acts of relational excellence, and by telling stories that foreground empathy, not just efficiency.

There is also a need for rituals that sustain moral clarity. Ethics rounds, patient story-sharing forums, and reflective debriefs can serve as anchors in high-pressure environments. These practices help teams pause and ask: *Are we still caring well? What does good look like here—not just efficient, but humane?*

Resisting Dehumanisation Is Not Nostalgia

It is tempting to frame the call for more humane institutions as a defence of tradition against technology. But that is a false binary. The issue is not whether AI belongs in healthcare—it already does, and it will only deepen. The question is: *On what terms?* Who gets to decide what is implemented, how it is used, and what success looks like?

Building institutions that resist dehumanisation is not about rejecting progress; it is about defining it. It is about ensuring that our enthusiasm for innovation does not outrun our capacity for wisdom. It is about recognising that care is not merely a transaction or a technical intervention—it is a human practice, grounded in trust, shaped by context, and accountable to meaning.

This is not an idealistic aspiration—it is a practical necessity. Systems that ignore human dignity are not merely unkind; they are unstable. Distrust grows where people feel invisible. Burnout escalates where workers are treated as inputs. And harm increases where complexity is reduced to codes.

We do not need perfect institutions. But we urgently need courageous ones—institutions willing to name and navigate the tensions between technological capability and ethical responsibility. Ones that will invest in governance that sees further, education that thinks deeper, and cultures that care better.

In the end, the future of humane healthcare will not be written in code, but in choices—policies crafted with moral clarity, clinicians trained in ethical discernment, and systems designed not merely for output, but for meaning. The task before us is not simply to keep pace with innovation. It is to shape it wisely—on human terms.

The Reader's Role in the System

The future of healthcare is not being written in code alone. It is being shaped, quietly but decisively, by the expectations, demands, and voices of those who participate in the system—patients, professionals, and policymakers alike. Amid the accelerating adoption of artificial intelligence in clinical settings, the prevailing narrative often casts individuals as passive recipients of innovation. But this framing is both strategically flawed and ethically hollow. The real power—and responsibility—lies not in the machines, but in the humans who choose how those machines are developed, deployed, and governed. The reader, in other words, is not a bystander. They are a stakeholder.

AI in medicine is not an autonomous evolution. It is the result of deliberate design decisions, shaped by values, incentives, and institutional dynamics. And because those decisions affect the moral texture of care—how we diagnose, treat, and relate to one another—they cannot be left to technologists alone. Nor should they. Every individual who touches the system, from a clinician consulting a decision-support algorithm to a patient consenting to AI-driven screening, participates in shaping its future. *Ethics does not reside upstream in the laboratory; it emerges downstream in use, friction, and feedback.* To reclaim ethical agency in this moment requires more than good intentions. It demands critical literacy, practical tools, and the courage to speak into systems that often feel too complex to question.

At the heart of this subchapter is a provocation: What does it mean for a reader to become an active agent in the design and governance of AI in healthcare? This is not an abstract philosophical prompt. It's a pragmatic challenge with real implications—on how clinicians evaluate the tools presented to them, on how patients negotiate choices framed by algorithms, and on how institutions cultivate environments that foreground care over compliance. Each of these roles requires its own strategies, language, and mode of engagement. Yet all share a common premise: *ethical systems are sustained not by rules alone, but by recurring moments of courageous conversation.*

For clinicians, reclaiming interpretive authority means learning how to challenge algorithmic recommendations—not from a place of hostility, but from a stance of informed curiosity. What was this model trained on? What does it assume about risk, value, and outcome? When does it fail, and for whom? Such questions are not technical distractions; they are clinical necessities. The art of medicine has always involved the navigation of ambiguity. But when algorithms appear to collapse uncertainty into probabilities and options into recommendations, the clinician's interpretive role becomes both more critical and more fragile. A powerful strategy is to develop routines of algorithmic interrogation—practices that incorporate questioning into standard workflows. Just as differential diagnosis involves asking, "What else could this be?", AI-supported care must ask, "What does this system know, and what is it blind to?" The language here matters. We are not rejecting AI; we are re-situating it as an input—not an oracle.

For patients, the challenge is different. Few arrive at the clinic with a background in data science or a fluency in algorithmic logic. But they are no less entitled to transparency, and no less capable of advocating for dignity in care. One of the most powerful tools available to patients is *the well-framed question.* When confronted with a treatment option informed by AI, a patient might ask: "How was this recommendation determined?" or "Has this system been tested on people like me?" These are not confrontational questions; they are clarity-seeking. They assert the patient's right to understand—not in technical detail, but in ethical substance—what guides the choices before them. Equipping patients with scripts for these moments is not paternalistic. It is empowering. Just as informed consent is central to clinical ethics, *informed engagement must become central to AI ethics.*

Policy professionals and institutional leaders play a third, equally vital role. They are the stewards of systemic accountability—the ones who decide what is regulated, what is measured, and what is incentivised. Yet policy is rarely proactive; it tends to follow scandals, not anticipate them. Readers in these positions must learn to ask *not just whether a tool works, but for whom, at what cost, and by whose values.* An AI system that improves average outcomes while worsening disparities is not an innovation—it is a regression masked in statistical performance. To push for better design, these stakeholders need evaluative frameworks that go beyond efficiency or cost-savings. They must demand transparency audits, community consultation, and human-centred impact assessments as prerequisites for deployment. They must advocate for "algorithmic stewardship" roles within hospitals—intermediaries who can interpret, monitor, and mediate the use of AI tools at the bedside.

But systemic change cannot rely solely on individual action. Institutional support is required to normalise ethical questioning. Hospitals should train staff not only in how to use AI tools, but in how to push back against them. Medical schools should teach interpretive scepticism alongside statistical reasoning. Patient advocacy groups should develop literacy programmes that decode technical jargon into accessible guidance. The ecosystem must evolve to protect the *right to understand* as vigorously as it protects the *right to privacy.*

What all of this demands is a shift in mindset. The ethical life of a technology does not begin and end in its design; it lives in the relationships it mediates. That means every reader of this book—whether they prescribe, receive, legislate, or simply fund care—has a role to play. You don't need to be an ethicist to raise ethical concerns. You don't need to be a programmer to question programming. You simply need to take seriously the proposition that *good technology is not what works—it is what aligns with the values we refuse to compromise.*

To that end, the following pages offer a repertoire of questions, scripts, and strategies. These are not checklists to memorise, but tools to adapt. Think of them as conversational scaffolding—structures that support better dialogue between humans and the systems they co-create. For clinicians, they provide phrasing to reassert judgement amid statistical certainty. For patients, they supply language to clarify and affirm personhood. For policymakers, they offer a lexicon of ethical scrutiny that resists reduction to metrics.

This is where the transformation begins—not with new code or more powerful models, but with readers who refuse to settle for systems that reduce care to calculus. The future of healthcare is not waiting to be discovered. *It is waiting to be demanded.*

Imagining the Next Era of Care

The future of healthcare will not be engineered solely through faster algorithms or more data points. It will be judged by its capacity to restore something older, more fragile, and far harder to quantify: care itself. For decades, technological innovation in medicine has rightly focused on scale, speed, and survival—moving us from crude diagnostics to precision therapies, from reactive medicine to predictive analytics. Yet as we now enter an age defined by artificial intelligence, machine learning, and ambient surveillance, the most urgent question is not what more we can measure—but what we might stop noticing. *The next era of care will hinge not on how much information machines can process, but on whether the systems we build can still hold a human story with dignity.*

It is easy to mistake intelligence for wisdom, and decision support for decision sufficiency. Today's AI models can detect diabetic retinopathy with startling accuracy, analyse CT scans faster than any radiologist, and recommend treatment pathways from terabytes of patient data. These feats are impressive and often lifesaving. But they do not, on their own, make a system worthy of trust. A predictive tool can flag a cardiac risk in milliseconds—but cannot discern whether the patient sitting across the room fears hospitals, values quality over longevity, or grieves the loss of a loved one. *Data can approximate risk; it cannot surface meaning.*

If the last decade has been about digitising medicine, the next must be about rehumanising it. This means designing systems that do not treat human values as "soft" data, or patient preferences as downstream from the algorithm, but rather place these perspectives at the centre of care. It means building tools that amplify—not supplant—the interpretive capacities of clinicians. And it means holding on to the radical proposition that care is not just a service or a protocol, but a relationship.

The philosophical shift is subtle but profound: away from viewing patients as data subjects to be optimised, and toward recognising them as persons to be understood. The logic of technological progress tends to favour abstraction. Patients become datasets. Clinicians become workflow nodes. Outcomes become metrics to be compared and managed. In such a frame, uncertainty is seen as an inefficiency, and individual complexity as noise. But real care often begins in the unmeasurable—when a physician listens just a little longer, or a nurse adjusts a protocol to preserve a patient's dignity.

To build this future, we must first name the gap between technological capability and ethical design. Many healthcare institutions now implement AI systems with little clarity around accountability: Who is responsible when an algorithm recommends an inappropriate treatment? What counts as informed consent when the underlying model is a black box? When predictive tools flag someone as "high risk," do patients have the right to contest the categorisation—or to refuse being profiled at all? *These are not peripheral questions. They are central to the legitimacy of any future healthcare system.*

A framework for ethical integration must therefore begin with three imperatives. First, *accountability*: every system should have a clear trail of responsibility, not just for its outputs but for how those outputs are used in clinical settings. Second, *explainability*: patients and clinicians alike must be able to understand—at an appropriate level—how a system arrives at its recommendations. And third, *human alignment*: no matter how efficient a system becomes, it should always be evaluated against its alignment with human values, autonomy, and cultural context. A system that can optimise drug dosages across millions of records but cannot honour a patient's end-of-life wishes is, by definition, misaligned.

But ethical frameworks alone will not be sufficient unless embedded in institutions capable of resisting dehumanisation. This will require cultural as well as technical transformation. Medical education must shift from teaching students to "follow the protocol" to equipping them to interpret, mediate, and challenge algorithmic outputs. Policies must be developed that preserve human judgment as a check on machine logic—not as a formality but as a core safeguard. Hospitals and clinics must actively measure not just throughput or patient satisfaction, but whether their technologies reinforce or erode the conditions of care: trust, time, and attentiveness.

Crucially, the responsibility to shape this future cannot rest with technologists or ethicists alone. Readers—whether patients, practitioners, educators, or policymakers—play a pivotal role. Asking better questions at the point of care can be transformative. Patients can ask, "Was this recommendation generated by a machine? What other options are possible?" Clinicians can ask, "Does this tool serve the patient's values—or just institutional targets?" Policymakers can ask, "Whose interests are embedded in the design of this system—and who was at the table when it was built?" *Care is too important to be delegated to code without scrutiny.*

Imagining the next era of care is not a speculative exercise. The early outlines are already here. Community health workers using voice-based AI tools to support patients in low-literacy environments. Hospital systems embedding patient narratives directly into clinical decision interfaces. Mental health platforms offering asynchronous care that still manages to feel deeply personal. These are not perfect solutions, but they gesture toward something vital: technology that bends to the complexity of the human condition, rather than flattening it.

The path forward is neither a return to nostalgic humanism nor blind embrace of automation. It is a third path—deliberate, careful, and designed with humility. One in which *data is not discarded but contextualised, systems are not rejected but shaped, and care is not lost but reclaimed.* The future of healthcare, if it is to be worthy of the name, must not simply ask what is possible. It must insist on asking: *what matters?* And who gets to decide?

About the Author

Elias Wren is a writer and systems thinker drawn to the places where innovation collides with human complexity. His work explores how technology reshapes the most intimate dimensions of life—health, identity, and care—often faster than our ethics can follow. With a background spanning design research, cultural analysis, and digital policy advising, Wren writes to equip readers with insight, not certainty. His writing is driven by a simple conviction: better systems begin with better questions. Beyond Precision reflects years of listening to patients, clinicians, and technologists grappling with what it really means to personalize care in an age of algorithms.

www.ingramcontent.com/pod-product-compliance
Lightning Source LLC
Chambersburg PA
CBHW031341230926
51848CB00002B/334
9789371770439